Chic & Slim
ENCORE

MORE
ABOUT HOW
FRENCH WOMEN
DRESS CHIC
STAY SLIM
—AND HOW
YOU CAN TOO

Anne Barone

THE ANNE BARONE COMPANY

Chic & Slim ENCORE:
More About How French Women Dress Chic Stay Slim
—and How You Can Too
Anne Barone

ISBN: 978-1-937066-03-1
A Chic & Slim Book
Published by The Anne Barone Company, Texas 76309 USA

Third Edition
Book Cover & Design: Anne Barone
Chic Woman Image Copyright © iStockphoto/karrapa
Eiffel Tower Design: Joyce Wells *GriggsArt*

This book is intended as philosophy and general reference only. It is not to be used as a substitute for medical advice or treatment. Every individual's problems with excess weight are unique and complex. You should consult your physician for guidance on any medical condition or health issue and to make certain any products or treatments you use are right and safe for you. The author and publisher disclaim any responsibility for any liability, loss or risk incurred directly or indirectly from the use or application of any of the contents of this publication or from any of the materials, services or products mentioned in the contents of this book or in supplemental materials published on the supporting website *annebarone.com*.

Readers Praise Chic & Slim

One For Me And One For Mom

I just wanted to thank you for writing such a wonderful little book. I immediately bought a copy for my mother and told two people at work about it. Your book is a rare find and so appreciated by someone who knows intrinsically that food is a wonderful part of life meant to be enjoyed and not abused or used to punish ourselves. — **Jill**

Weight Loss Success

I've adopted a number of your diet tips, along with some others that I think "mesh" with my personality and lifestyle. I've lost 5 of my ten pounds...I have more energy lately to boot! All this and I don't have to give up my daily cup of coffee and my nightly glass of wine. *C'est formidable*, Madame! *Merci!* —**Karen in Cleveland**

Just Wonderful

What's so wonderful about what you're doing is I'm a Francophile. I love fashion, beauty, and decorating (in the words of CNN's Elsa Klensch). I love to cook. I want to stay slim. I want to enjoy life in the way the Europeans seem to enjoy life, and rather than trying to chase down each of those threads independently, your web page and book incorporate all of those things into a single source. Every part of the book and website captures some part of a lifestyle that interests me both intellectually and aesthetically. They're just wonderful!!
— Marsi in Denver

Better Way

Thank you for *Chic&Slim*. I've almost got it memorized after several readings. It's a much better way to spend the evening than checking what might be in the kitchen whispering my name. — **AD**

Thank you

Thank you for what you are doing for American women!
— Ruth in Boston

this book is dedicated
to all those

CHIC&SLIM WOMEN

whose enthusiasm
for the original *Chic&Slim:
how those chic French women
eat all that rich food
and still stay slim*
and for the *Chic&Slim* website
annebarone.com
inspired this book

CONTENTS

About Author Anne Barone

Once fat and frumpy, in her mid-20s Anne Barone began to learn chic French women's techniques for eating well and staying slim and for dressing chic on a small budget. She lost 55 pounds and acquired a chic French wardrobe. Chicer and slimmer, Anne Barone returned to the USA to find a nation growing sloppier and fatter. She decided to share her French secrets.

In 1997, Anne Barone published her first French-inspired book *Chic&Slim: how those chic French women eat all that rich food and still stay slim.* More *Chic&Slim* books followed.

In her books and on the *Chic&Slim* companion website *annebarone.com*, Anne Barone continues to share French secrets for dressing chic and staying slim.

Now 67, Anne Barone lives in Texas where she is attempting to create a bit of French Provence on the North Texas plains. "Far enough in the country to grow eggplant, apricots and lavender. But close enough to Dallas to make the sales at Neiman Marcus."

rode her bicycle until she was 100 and continued to walk regularly even after giving up cycling. But most important, they felt, Jeanne Calment seemed to have a natural immunity to stress. More likely, early in her life, she had developed an effective means of coping with stress. One thing you so often notice about French women is that air of serenity they carry about them.

An American writer living in France, Marianne Jacobbi, observed of the French: "They know that to stay fit for life you have to do more than restrict your diet or go for the burn: You have to pamper your soul. French culture revolves around the principle that stress subtracts years from your life and pleasure prolongs it."

When the French sit around in cafés, they aren't doing nothing. They are practicing stress therapy.

LES NOUVEAUX PURITANS

When the French find Americans doing something that surprises or perplexes them, they often chalk it up to *le puritanisme*. On the matter of pleasure, the attitudinal gulf between the two nationalities gapes as wide as the Atlantic Ocean our early American forebears crossed to establish their religious colonies in the New World.

Those *Mayflower* passengers may have long lain beneath their unadorned New England tombstones, but they have left us with a Puritan legacy that, though it has undergone modification and mutation over the centuries, still colors American thinking and lifestyle. And when Americans actually do something pleasurable, the action often generates a quantity of guilt sufficiently weighty that, loaded in the cargo hold, it would have sunk the *Mayflower* before it sailed from its English port.

PURITAN THINKING

To the Puritan way of thinking, anything that brings pleasure is bad. Discomfort and sacrifice are good. The more uncomfortable and unpleasant something is, the better the Puritans think it is for us. Having failed to stamp out sex, and no longer convincing the majority of Americans that card playing, seeing movies, wearing makeup, and dancing are the road to damnation, American Puritanism has undergone an evolution. Nouveaux Puritans no longer preach against pleasure for moral or religious reasons, now they have drawn up a whole new list of no-nos on the principle that such things are bad for our health. Eating takes the brunt of their attack.

The Nouveaux Puritans don't want anyone to eat anything that tastes good without paying a price. And they certainly don't want us to lose weight and stay slim unless we suffer a rigid regime of tasteless, unappetizing food. They would prefer, I think, that we endure hunger pains at least six hours a day in order to stay slim and healthy.

Nouveaux Puritans do not think much of Anne Barone's French-inspired *Chic&Slim* philosophy. I witnessed an excellent demonstration of this Nouveau Puritan attitude at a book signing. Among the *Chic&Slim* promotional materials was that phrase I often use: *The French eat chocolate, cheese, and pastry and still stay slim. And you can too.* This phrase so infuriated one man who read it that he demanded that I take down the poster. "It's a lie," he bellowed at me, his finger shaking at the offending words.

Well, it wasn't a lie. Standing there, I was living, breathing proof that you could eat chocolate, cheese, and pastry and still stay slim. But I learned years ago it wastes breath to argue with a fanatic. So I remained cool and diplomatic. (Though I actually thought the man was a bad combination of rude and loony.) Eventually he ran out of steam and went on his way. About 15 minutes later, he was back.

This Nouveau Puritan was now telling me how to lose weight. He sounded like Dr. Dean Ornish in a really strict mood. Limit fats to 10 percent of daily calories, no red meat, no butter, no this, no that. So much exercise per day. You know the drill.

Did he actually follow this program he was outlining?

Well, no. He was 50, maybe more, pounds overweight, with his big belly bulging out his Hawaiian shirt. And there I was, the 55-year-old Ms. Chocolate, Cheese & Pastry in her slim straight skirt, beginning to become a little annoyed with this character. I have certainly never

ATTITUDE TOWARD EFFORT

Another major difference between US and French cultures I observed is the attitude toward effort. Post-World War II American culture in which I grew up put much emphasis on labor-saving devices and instant foods, mixes, processed foods, and frozen TV dinners. The intention was well-meaning. Especially during frontier days and the Great Depression, life in the United States was so filled with deprivation and drudgery, particularly for women, that things such as cake mixes, instant pudding, frozen dinners, electric mixers, automatic washing machines and clothes dryers were viewed in the 1950s as true gifts to make women's lives easier. Compensatory payment for those years of deprivation and drudgery. Not long ago my mother commented on making an angel food cake as a teenager without so much as a wire whisk, much less a mixer. She whipped those dozen egg whites by hand with two forks.

By the early 1960s, when Julia Child introduced Americans to the art of French cooking, most American cookbooks were filled with recipes that called for a package of instant this and a bottle of prepared something else. When the Peace Corps began in 1961, the compilers of the Peace Corps book locker had a difficult time finding an American cookbook to include. Peace Corps Volunteers would serve in countries where instants and mixes were unavailable. They finally chose an edition of Fanny Farmer's *Boston Cooking School Cookbook* as the one whose recipes relied less on mixes and prepared ingredients.

EFFORT FOR PLEASURE

In an *Elle Decor* article, chic French woman Katell Le Bourhis, a protégé of fashion legend Diana Vreeland, catalogs all the efforts that go into her personal style including washing and ironing the cocktail napkins for her guests. "I love the effort," she says.

Many Americans have lost touch with the satisfaction of the effort. They are always looking for ways to avoid it. But in avoiding the effort, they often miss some real pleasure. Some of those pleasure-producing efforts would fill up some of the time they now devote to overeating.

I discovered early that French women did not seem to mind the effort. They cooked from scratch. In those days, every French woman I knew had a kitchen with far fewer appliances and gadgets than American women did. Plumbing often fell into a category that could be described as antiquated. Refrigerators and cooking ranges were generally much smaller than American models. Often half the size or less. Some kitchens had no cooking stove, only a hot plate, sometimes a double hot plate attached to bottled gas. But I never heard French women complain about how hard it was to prepare a meal on these appliances. They seemed to take pleasure from their efforts because those efforts produced results that pleased them. They demonstrated this attitude not only toward food preparation, but to their appearance as well.

One young French woman I knew dressed herself on an impossibly limited budget. She made all her dresses by hand. I have sat and chatted with her as she made tiny stitches in fabric with her needle. I must say, though, that I was not terribly surprised when she told me her hobby was nudism.

Every year she and her husband took their month of August vacation at a nudist colony. If I had to sew all my clothes by hand, I, too, might adopt nudism as a hobby. As it was, it certainly seemed to solve the problem of packing. Stick your toothbrush and a comb in your purse and away you go.

The French believe that effort brings better results and consequently heightens pleasure. So the effort is worth it, because it increases their *joie de vivre*. Americans believe that labor-saving appliances and products save them work, and consequently they have more pleasure because they have more leisure.

Something that occurred while I was writing this book contributed to my thinking on the difference in the American and French attitudes toward effort. I was in the natural foods store, dipping organic soy flour out of the bin, when another shopper asked me what I did with soy flour. I explained I was putting more soy in my diet because of numerous proven health benefits, especially for women. Of the variety of ways I was including it in my daily eating, was that I substituted a cup of soy flour for one of whole wheat in my breakfast bread recipe.

She wasn't interested in soy flour, but she wanted me to try her favorite product. It was a muffin mix. "Our doctor limits us to 30 percent fat in our diet," she said. She gestured toward her husband, a generously proportioned male senior citizen poking into other bins down the aisle. "We give ourselves a treat," she went on holding up a bag containing yellowish powder infested with small purple nodules. "This blueberry muffin mix is so easy. You only have to add water and stir."

I bit my tongue to keep from telling her that I ate a healthy low-fat diet (because I eat a lot of fresh veggies and fruits). When I wanted a treat, I could certainly come up with something better than a tasteless mix containing fake fruit. There was at that moment a beautiful display of fresh, delicious Texas blueberries in the produce section of the store. Why not buy a package and make a lovely blueberry muffin in which you could reduce the fat to a far lower level than what was in that mix she was buying? I have been making muffins for years with a quarter or less of the amount of oil called for in your typical muffin recipe.

A problem of time-saving mixes (beyond inferior taste) is that you spend less time on preparation. Quick preparation leaves you with a *lot* of time for eating. Especially for eating that second helping you don't really need. Not only was this woman fat, she was that flabby kind of fat that comes when you don't get the proper amount of physical exercise. She was living, walking proof of the reports that as Americans have cut their fat consumption, they have substituted in refined carbohydrates and sugar as in "low-fat" bakery products such as this muffin mix with its white flour, sugar, and fakey purple things substituted for real fruit.

WANTED: SILVER BULLETS

In the USA, any weight control product that successfully defines itself as a "silver bullet" becomes very popular. (Usually commercially successful in addition.) One product that became very popular was in the form of bars that were marketed to those following the Dr. Atkins' high-protein weight control program. A woman who worked in a store that sold these supplements said that for a time they could not keep them in stock.

Why were the supplements so popular? Her answer: "People want things prepared. They want something they can grab and take with them."

At one point, when all the Dr. Atkins' supplements were sold out, she said some customers who came to the store to purchase them became almost frantic. She suggested that if they wanted to lose weight, supplements weren't really necessary. It was just a matter of eating a bit less and exercising a bit more. "But people do not want to hear that," she said. "They want to take a pill and not have to worry about putting out any effort."

They also do not want to make any lifestyle changes.

Supplements might help you lose weight short-term. But if you are overweight, likely you will have to make some changes in your lifestyle and your eating habits if you want to live as slim as the French on a permanent basis. "Does that mean I have to start wearing a turtleneck, a beret, sexy lingerie and high heels?" one woman asked me.

Finding your own personal silver bullet might be easier than you think. Often no major overhaul of lifestyle is needed. All that is required is to identify the *one* thing that is putting an excess of calories in your daily food intake. If you can substitute something else for that one thing, often over time, you will experience a steady loss of excess weight until you reach a normal weight. In the original *Chic & Slim*, I related how singer Reba McEntire had credited her weight loss to substituting mineral water for the beer she had been in the habit of drinking.

Often, awareness can solve your excess weight problem. At a seminar, a woman in her late forties asked for advice about a baffling weight gain of 20 pounds over the past two years. She was eating and exercising exactly the same as she had all her adult life when she had easily maintained a normal weight. We talked a bit. She told me since the time her children were small, she had worked full time plus led an active social life.

What struck me as I listened to her describe her life was that she now had time to finish her meals in leisure. When I told her this, she thought a moment, then, she told me she realized that she was actually eating second helpings because for the first time in a couple of decades she had time for them.

Two months later, Helen phoned me and told me she had just had her checkup with her doctor. She had lost 11 of the 20 pounds she needed to lose. She said she had not made any particular effort at weight loss, certainly she had not followed a "diet." She had simply been aware of her previous unconscious overeating. She now stopped eating when her hunger was satisfied, rather than when the serving bowls on the dinner table were empty.

Without a doubt, women living in France have an easier time staying slim than women who live in many other countries, particularly women who live in the United States. The USA is surely the most difficult location in the world for maintaining a normal weight.

Women in France have the advantage of living in a culture that makes staying slim easily possible. On the other hand, American culture makes maintaining a normal weight very difficult.

At this point, if you are on your way to the nearest French Consulate to apply for a long-term visa, that's not necessary. With the information in this book, you can achieve that French state of chic and slim no matter where you live.

Now that you have a background on culture, you need to understand how French women and their efforts in *"l'art de femme,"* their art of being women, is crucial in their efforts to stay chic and slim.

PRAISE FOR CHIC & SLIM WEBSITE
annebarone.com

Dear Anne,

I cannot express how greatly I enjoy visiting your website, and it's a rare phenomenon indeed to find one so assiduously updated. I really look forward to going there on what has become almost a daily ritual! I get the same satisfaction as I do from reading my Paris Vogue, watching an Audrey Hepburn film, or having a lovely glass of soft merlot. I feel so 'at home', I cannot describe this feeling any better than that! I love your philosophy, and commonsense tips, along with your France links and the afternoon teas are an inspiration.

I wish to say *merci beaucoup* to you for a taste of French culture and style that transcends mere dietary considerations. You have a holistic approach that is not puritanical nor does it emphasize unrealistic modifications. It is so easy to integrate your ideas into a full and busy life.

— ***Antoinette in Australia***

a few *faux pas*. Everyone does. Some who made the worst mistakes in the beginning turned out splendidly elegant later. One thinks of Diana, Princess of Wales, and some of those unflattering outfits in which she was photographed during the first years after her marriage to Prince Charles. But she learned. Before her death, she developed a personal style in which she looked marvelous whether she was wading through a minefield in jeans or dining at a state dinner in a formal evening gown.

We must accept that in developing and evolving our personal styles we will occasionally make a choice that will not turn out right. We need to develop that capacity French women have for accepting those mistakes as part of the process. And never, ever admit that we made a mistake. (*Moi?* Mistake? *Pas possible!*) It is also useful to know the address of a good resale shop.

WHAT IS THEIR MOTIVATION?

Perfecting their art of being women takes time and energy. Developing a chic, workable personal style isn't something that happens without thought and effort. Why are French women willing to spend hours, weeks, months, years deciding exactly what style looks best on them? Why are they content to spend so much time deciding which lipstick shade is the most flattering to their skin tone, or selecting a *parfum* that best expresses their personality? Why do French women take all that time to iron their clothes into smooth perfection, budget for facials, save for months, even years to buy one designer handbag, spend a week in a spa undergoing sea water spray from a high pressure hose? Why do they torture their toes with impossibly high heeled shoes when a pair of flats or sneakers would be more comfortable?

French women design a personal style so that they will be attractive and alluring to men. French women want male admiration and attention; they want affection. If a few little gifts are offered, that's nice too. In the USA, a man offering an admiring compliment to a woman runs the risk of being yelled at, slapped, even sued for harassment. If he pays a compliment in the workplace, he might face disciplinary action.

American women are insulted if they are considered a sex object.

In France, a woman is insulted if she is NOT considered an object of desire. The compliment, the admiring male glance, the whistle, the occasional pat, the whispered suggestions: these serve as confirmation that a French woman is succeeding as a woman.

USEFUL ATTRACTIVE APPEARANCE

French women find an attractive appearance an advantage not just in social situations, but also in the workplace, in shopping, and in coping with bureaucrats. That is not to suggest that they are bestowing sexual favors in return for promotions, better service or telephone repair. But men are visually oriented. Business presentations can often be boring: an overhead projector throwing bar graphs on a screen quickly becomes about as scintillating as looking at a friend's out-of-focus vacation photos. How much more tolerable the presentation if the woman showing the bar graph slides has a shapely leg, or a skirt that shapes around a nice derrière. How much more pleasant for the shop clerk or the telephone repairman if Madame has an interesting face, or if her sweater clings in just the right way.

MÈRE & FILLE, GRAND-MÈRE & PETITE-FILLE

In matters of personal style and techniques of weight control, French women have another advantage over American women: their mothers. Those of us who had mothers who were overweight and who taught us or allowed us to develop bad food habits are at a disadvantage.

In a Mexican restaurant, I observed an incident involving an American grandmother and an overweight granddaughter. A good example of how often overweight American women do not receive the helpful guidance French mothers and grandmothers dispense to their daughters and granddaughters.

The waitress brought tortillas. Since this was a traditional Mexican family restaurant, those tortillas not only had a liberal amount of fat, but most likely it was *manteca*. The word is much prettier in Spanish than its English equivalent: lard.

The grandmother called the waitress. "She has to have butter."

these pricey glasses might be broken, I had horrible visions of spikes of shattered crystal slicing arteries in little wrists. "But she must learn," was my friend's response to my voiced worries.

In the USA, we give little hands non-breakable cups with easy-to-grasp handles. Usually with lids. We set them at tables with scratch-resistant, water-repellent surfaces, lest they dribble or spill. My friend's daughter's little fingers were barely able to stretch around the crystal tumbler on which the chilled fruit juice had beaded slippery moisture. She sat quietly at the table, using both hands to slowly convey the heavy glass to her little lips. She took care not to drop the glass or spill the liquid down on the surface of the polished mahogany table. She was learning the habit of sipping beverages in a polite manner. (Meanwhile I, watching, was an absolute nervous wreck.)

I served my child in Tupperware. My friend served her child in Baccarat. By the way, at Christmas I received a photo of that little girl now grown up a slim, chic, beautiful university graduate. I am sure she has lovely table manners.

FRENCH WOMEN: ARE THEY SNOBS?

French women, particularly Parisian women, have a reputation with Americans as snobbish, haughty. I always say in their defense that this was never my experience with French women. The only occasion in which a French woman acted in a rude manner toward me (when I had not inadvertently done something to provoke her rudeness) was in Strasbourg in the late 1970s. Strasbourg lies on the far eastern side of France near the German border in an area that has passed back and forth between German and French control. As in the Balkans, some present-day prejudices and animosities find their root in long-past historical events. I accompanied a German friend to an exclusive children's shop in downtown Strasbourg. My German friend asked the assistance of one of the French shop clerks. The other French woman clerk fastened me in a searing glare and began to hurl a stream of insults at me. Though I had not spoken, when she had heard my friend's German-accented French, she evidently assumed I, too, was German.

My French was sufficiently *au courant* I understood completely the depth of scorn the French woman was heaping on me. I said nothing, I simply gave the woman a contemptuous look as if I thought she was utterly out of her mind. Whether she shut up because of my acid look, because she had run out of anti-German bile, or because she decided on second glance that I was not German, I do not know.

A COMMENT ON SNOBBISH

As a friend who lived years in France and observed French women commented: "With regard to the setting of boundaries and appearing aloof and snobbish, I think French women allow themselves time to assess a given situation. This can appear to be aloofness or snobbishness. In fact, this allows them to be very serene and calm in any given situation. Very often elsewhere, people react first and think later."

How true.

When I was a child growing up in the United States, we were admonished by parents and teachers to think before we spoke. Now the model seems to be that everyone reacts immediately to their *feelings*. Everyone screams their immediate emotional reaction, rather than taking a moment to think, and, after thought, react in a reasonable manner. The benefit of giving ourselves time to assess a situation before reacting is preserving for ourselves that serenity and calmness that has so many benefits for French women. Including the benefit of helping keep them slim.

SOMETIMES DESERVED

I never observed an instance in which a French woman (or man) behaved frostily or in a rude manner toward an American in which the American had not provoked that rudeness by doing something considered impolite in French culture or that violated one of those rules of French behavior that guide the ritualized, tidy manner of French living.

If I was able to interact amicably with French women over the years, it may have, in some part, been the result of the environment in which I grew up. In that small town, many of our neighbors and

In Diane Johnson's award-nominated novel *Le Divorce*, the French husband's family does not fault him for divorcing his American wife. After all, she does not keep her nails well manicured. She is caring for a small child and pregnant and wears low-heeled shoes. Unsightly fingernails. Clunky shoes. Perfectly normal, to the French way of thinking, that the husband should have found another woman.

THAT STUNNING ACCESSORY

Because French women generally prefer small, workable wardrobes, they get great mileage out of accessories. Sometimes their choice of accessories are, well, unusual. Often what makes a chic French woman extraordinarily chic is not a scarf or belt or piece of jewelry, but something furry. I am not talking about mink or sable. The most unforgettably elegant French woman I ever saw was wearing a camel-colored wool pant suit, brown leather boots, and carrying a plain brown leather shoulder bag. Very nice, but nothing extraordinary. But elegantly positioned on a leash beside her was a sleek Afghan hound, as tall and slender as she, whose gleaming coat was a shade slightly darker than the woman's suit.

The dog was the coordinated accessory that made the French woman unforgettable. In my mind, I can still see that elegant woman and her elegant dog vividly these three decades later.

FRENCH CHIC IS NEAT

In almost every case when I have analyzed a French woman's chic, I rarely failed to notice neatness. Here is another factor. French women iron. Who has time to iron? you ask. French women make time to iron. (See the chapter on household organization for how they find time.) Need I point out that if you are ironing you are not lounging in front of the television nibbling high-calorie snacks?

After you study French women for a while, you realize how central a role neatness plays in their chic. This is especially true for women whose financial condition forces them to manage their chic on little money. A French woman will always buy "the best quality she can afford," but neatness makes it possible for many women who must dress with flea market finds and basics from Monoprix or Prix Unique (French versions of Walmart and Kmart) to look wonderful.

While I can understand how they have time to iron so they start out looking neat, what amazes me is how they manage to stay neat in so many circumstances that would rumple and wilt most of us in two minutes. Here's an example of what I mean. I made this observation on the Caribbean island of Martinique, as much a part of France as Hawaii is part of the United States. I had gone with a friend who spoke no French to the marina to serve as interpreter during the arrangements for a diving boat charter. The young French woman in charge of such matters was dressed in shorts and a cotton print top. They were, of course, both marvelously unwrinkled, and her short sleek hairdo flipped smartly below her ears. Someone unfamiliar with French women would have assumed that she had only arrived at the boat having recently dressed in fresh clothes and her hair had only seconds before had careful styling. I knew this was not the case.

The marina where the young woman worked was lined with shops and cafes I frequented regularly during my visit. She was there at her post from early morning until sundown. There in the sunny heat and humid wind of the marina, she remained wrinkle free, showing no signs of perspiration, and with neat hair no matter what time of day I saw her. She wore the same pair of dark khaki shorts, though her cool cotton tops varied from day to day.

Buying quality and insisting on perfect fit pays off. Clothes of high quality that fit you perfectly will withstand the rigors of climate and activity better than cheap clothes that don't fit well. That's why for travel you are smarter to buy one basic good quality outfit than divide the money for the purchase of three outfits of lesser quality.

STAYING NEAT

Beyond quality and fit, those ultrachic French women will, at times, go to extraordinary lengths to preserve their neatness. One evening many years ago, when I was first living abroad, I was invited to the apartment of a friend for a small *soirée*. The group of seven or eight women turned out to be multinational: French, German, British, and one woman of indeterminate nationality. I seem to remember I was the only American.

My friend served wine, cheese, bread, a platter of *crudités*, and some sweet biscuits: food that would constitute for us our evening meal. I was next to last to arrive. The conversation in progress involved living quarters was my first lesson in how focused Europeans, for whom small living spaces are the norm, think in terms of the actual measurements.

It was during the apartment discussion that Gisèle arrived. I call her Gisèle not to protect her privacy, but that evening at my friend's apartment took place more than 30 years ago. I simply do not remember the woman's name.

She was the epitome of French chic. She was medium height, and not thin, but every ounce on her body was firm and in the right spot to give her a wonderful feminine form. The evening was warm and humid, but not a strand of her smooth blond hair was out of place. She wore spotless, perfectly pressed and creased white cotton slacks, a sleeveless white top and hand-tooled leather sandals. The creamy color of her outfit set off the marvelous coppery gold of her suntan and accented her eyes that were a striking opal blue.

Gisèle made the rounds of the group, giving each of us that quick, firm French handshake. Then she did something that puzzled me. She turned and surveyed the four corners of the room, and after a moment's hesitation, walked purposely toward a chair in a corner near a bookshelf. What she did next surprised me even more. She slipped her feet out of her sandals, unfastened the waistband of her slacks, and carefully took them off.

No one else in the room seemed to pay the least attention to this undressing. The amicable conversation continued without pause. Meanwhile, with great care, Gisèle straightened the slacks so that the creased legs were perfectly aligned. She carefully placed them over the back of the chair. Then, in her white cotton top and her bikini underpants, she joined the group.

A couple of hours later, when it was time to go home, Gisèle returned to the corner. She carefully put her slacks back on, gave us all a farewell handshake, and departed—looking as elegantly neat as the moment she had walked through the door.

I cornered my hostess. In answer to my question, she shrugged, not much interested by the question. "Gisèle often does that." (Note here the acceptance of non-standard behavior as "that is just what a person does.") But why did she take off her slacks at a social gathering? One possibility I had initially considered was sunburn, or perhaps a rash that made wearing the slacks on a warm evening uncomfortable. But I had ruled out sunburn and rash. Her golden tan was deep and obviously the result of many weeks in the sun. No hint of redness or rash. Further research revealed answers both practical and simple. Gisèle often wore white because the color accented magnificently her natural coloring and splendid suntan. But sitting in cotton slacks in the humid evening air would surely wrinkle them. *(Quelle horreur!)* She (or someone else) might spill a drop of wine on those beautiful white slacks. Food stains are not chic. So the most *logical* solution was simply to take off the slacks.

Did Gisèle remove clothing even when men were present? I asked my friend. Yes, that had occurred. Surprised, I had to remind myself that Europeans are generally more comfortable with their bodies than their American cousins. In all honesty, in her cotton top and bikini underpants, she was more covered than most of us were when we appeared on the beach in our standard French bikinis. I was also told, that *chez elle*, Gisèle dealt with the warm weather and eased the strain on laundry duties by simply wearing nothing at all.

ATTENTION TO DETAIL

Anyone who has observed the French are aware of the most minute attention to detail they give everything. This habit particularly fascinates American observers. From the way they fold a letter, to the way they arrange food on a serving platter, to the color of gloves for a particular coat, the French do things very precisely. One French friend comments on the difference in the way we type on a computer keyboard. I type at breakneck pace, making lots of errors, backspacing and deleting rapidly. She types precisely, going about the process methodically and carefully. She rarely makes a mistake. She dresses the same way.

FRENCH CHIC IS ORIGINAL

French chic invariably contains an element of originality. A chic French woman aims to create a *unique* personal style. (That is why designers look to the street and to chic resorts for fashion inspiration.) French women often create totally original combinations. Creativity has been defined as taking two or more familiar things and putting them together in a way that has never been done before. An elegant silk shirt with jeans or two watches on the same wrist. At one time, they were "not done." Then some chic woman showed that they could be put together in a way that looked wonderful.

In the 1980s, you saw chic French women wearing ordinary white cotton T-shirts (plain old American Hanes was a favored brand) with an elegant scarf knotted around their neck. American actors Marlon Brando and James Dean had taken white T-shirts out of the underwear category and made them popular outerwear. Women had been wearing elegant scarves for decades. Then someone got the idea of wearing them together, and they looked marvelous. Of course, you could sit in a Parisian sidewalk cafe and watch 100 chic women walk past wearing the white T-shirt and scarf combination, but each would manage to have added some element that made hers a bit different.

Holly Brubach writing in "In Fashion" in The New Yorker observed: "Frenchwomen, even when they're wearing the same shirt or carrying the same handbag, somehow succeed in looking one of a kind, usually by virtue of some small detail. Living in Paris, one comes to realize that there are an infinite number of ways to tie a scarf or comb one's hair."

FRENCH CHIC IS DARING

French chic often demonstrates daring. (Please understand that by daring, I do not mean obscene or trashy.) When Coco Chanel decided to design her "sports" clothes for women out of machine knitted jersey, the fabric had only been used before in work clothes for fishermen. Fashionable women had only worn real jewels. Coco Chanel had plenty of those, thanks to generous men in her life. But she made wearing fake or costume jewelry popular, and then dared to wear real and costume jewelry at the same time. That practice today is so common that few would find it unusual.

THE GREATEST GAME IN FRANCE

Choosing what to wear is never drudgery for French women. *La mode* is a game they have great fun playing. For this reason a chic French woman never looks dull or boring. She successfully gets our attention, and we enjoy what we see.

Along with seeing fashion as a game, the French give the same sort of attention to the seasonal fashion shows that Americans give to Super Bowl, and the World Series. Yet you must remember that there is a great difference between what a chic French woman wears and what is seen in the Paris fashion shows. Just as there is great difference in what the chicly dressed American woman wears and what some of our more avant-garde American designers send down the runway each season.

FASHION SHOWS AS THEATER

Given the French economy with its high unemployment, most French women must achieve their chic without couture dresses and designer ready-to-wear. The fashion shows we see on television and on *style.com* videos are theater. But entertaining theater, true.

A different sort of fashion theater can be very useful, as actress Isabella Rossellini explained to Michael Quintanilla, fashion writer of the *Los Angeles Times,* in an article "Fashion Is a Game We Play." Defining the difference between style and fashion, Isabella Rossellini said: "At home, fashion is individual theater. The way we dress up or the way women use makeup, that's our little theater on ourselves, a moment where we say, 'I'm a star.'" She believes that the benefits to playing this fashion theater game is that you will learn that fashion is an expression of your tastes and a reflection of what you like for yourself. "Style is an expression of one's self." Isabella Rossellini says fashion designers can stimulate your own ideas. Useful because it is difficult to develop your own personal style. She advises you to look to designers for ideas and inspiration for your own unique style.

For a woman who looks to the fashion shows to stimulate ideas for her own fashion, those theatrical extravaganzas might be entertaining, but not necessarily helpful. I wish more would be modeled on Betsey Johnson's Spring 2000 show. In an effort to show how her clothes looked on real people, the American designer forsook professional models and called on friends and family members of all ages and sizes to model her designs.

A chic French woman might follow media reports on fashion shows, but she would spend more time sitting in a sidewalk cafe watching the fashion show put on by real women.

FRENCH CHIC HAS SEXY ALLURE

While French chic is not obscene, French chic does have allure. It's sexy. But never in a trampy, trashy way. French chic somehow manages to be sensual, yet tasteful. Chic women are careful not to cross the line into bad taste. If you spend time observing them, you will see this is so. Writing a recipe for exactly how they accomplish sexy yet tasteful is more difficult.

This is where the reserve and propriety that often earns French women a reputation for being snobbish or haughty is useful to them. French women don't smile as much as American women. If they dressed in their alluring manner *and* flashed a warm smile at every stranger on the street, they likely would find themselves in real trouble.

If French women were friendly and outgoing to every chance acquaintance, a black leather skirt slit up the thigh and high-heel ankle strap sandals might send a more provocative message. That rather severe look many French women wear as the standard facial expression can intimidate. And protect.

The French do not make new friends readily. That French reserve is always at work. France is also an extremely class-conscious society.

People are hesitant to step across social boundaries. That distance, that invisible wall that French women seem to keep between them and all except their close acquaintances and their family, is useful. And protecting.

AUDREY, EXAMPLE OF RESERVE

Early in her career when actress Audrey Hepburn starred as a sea nymph in the Broadway play *Ondine*, the costume she wore was nothing more than a bit of fishnet to which seaweed had been attached in three or four strategic spots. This was the early 1950s when censorship in films and plays was strict. Sea nymphs and mermaids when played by the average glamorous Hollywood actress were usually costumed in a one-piece bathing suit of thick fabric and a from-the-waist-down fishtail with heavy scales. Yet no complaint was voiced against Audrey Hepburn's unusually revealing outfit. One writer's comment that I remember reading was that because Audrey was who she was, no one said a thing.

We have been assured by hundreds of her friends and coworkers that Audrey Hepburn was a deeply warm and caring person. But in her early years in Hollywood, she was considered snobbish and standoffish by many working in the film industry. What they were observing was that European reserve and caution in developing social relationships. These traits were probably even stronger in Audrey Hepburn than the average European woman. Her mother was a baroness. Her mother's sister was a lady-in-waiting to Queen Juliana of the Netherlands.

CIVIC DUTY

A French woman feels an obligation to show others her attractive appearance. Much in the same way a civic-minded American feels the obligation to keep the lawn mowed, home in good repair, and no trash allowed to collect around the house in order to keep their city and neighborhood attractive. A French woman knows that looking at an attractive, well-dressed woman is a pleasure. But looking at a woman with an unattractive personal style is not an aesthetically appealing experience. In France, much importance is placed on the appearance of a woman. In the United States, a man would impress other men by the kind of vehicle he drove or other possessions. In France, he might be more likely to be judged by the appearance of the woman with whom he is seen. Not just husbands and lovers, but the whole family would be shamed by a French woman's slovenliness. (In another part of the book, I recount how one nine-year-old boy was taunted by friends at school because his mother was overweight.)

This societal pressure to appear attractive puts pressure on a French woman to keep her weight under control and her *ligne* (form) svelte. We have pressures like this in the USA, but in different regions and in different socioeconomic groups, it is not as strong as in others. Consequently, in some geographic regions we find a larger percentage of the population that is overweight. Statistics show that, in general, the better educated and more affluent are more likely to be slim. The poor are more likely to be overweight.

CHIC EVERYWHERE

An interesting question came from a man who had spent several weeks traveling throughout France. Why was it that women living in rural areas in France maintain a chic, attractive appearance while many American women in rural areas do not achieve the levels of chic of their urban sisters?

(Please note that the following is my opinion based on observations over the years.) The whole country of France is only as big as Texas, one of the larger states of the USA. You don't find such a great difference in people in different regions and of different economic classes in that country. Additionally, the tendency toward neatness is very much a part of the French culture. As I've said previously, much of French chicness comes from plain old neatness.

France never had a frontier. American frontier women's lives were too difficult to leave much time for giving themselves the kind of care to look attractive. They were trying to survive, keep the family fed, and keep at least a few of the children they bore alive until their eighteenth birthday. Habits are passed from mother to daughter. Also, many of the immigrants were the poorest of peasants. These women had never had the leisure or the money to dress elegantly. Again, they did not have habits that were passed down mother-to-daughter.

One reason French women are always able to appear chic is that in France it is impolite to drop by a person's house uninvited. Since people don't drop by, a French woman can do her beauty maintenance and not worry about someone coming to the door interrupting hair coloring or a facial.

Another factor in French chicness, I am convinced, is the weather. France is on about the same latitude as the northernmost part of the USA. It is easier to look chic and neat if you aren't soaked in perspiration. Also, casual clothes for cooler climates tend to look neater than casual clothes for scorching climates.

And lastly, *le puritanisme* plays a role.

American rural areas often have populations with members of religious faiths that believe one should not put effort into looking attractive. A woman should be doing good works for the poor, or serving her church, not taking bubble baths and waxing her legs.

Often, women who dress the best in these areas are those of low morals. So a nice woman would hesitate to dress well for fear of looking as if she is out to seduce someone. Even if her religious beliefs do not have as strict a dress code as some of the sects, if those sects make up the majority of the population, a woman often dresses well at her peril.

In France, you can look chic and still be a nice, moral woman who simply has pride in her appearance. Even if a woman *is* out to seduce someone, that is not necessarily seen as evil.

KNOWING WHEN TO BREAK RULES

French chic knows when to break the rules. There have been times when I have seen a French woman wearing an outfit that I would never have dared wear for fear of looking odd. But they carry it off with such élan. They think they look wonderful and somehow they convince people who see them that they do look wonderful. I remember the

French woman I saw shopping. She had artfully tied a tablecloth into a sarong. It looked splendidly chic worn with sandals and gold hoop earrings.

THE BOTTOM LINE IS CONFIDENCE

Analyzing French chic, we consider French women's preferences for neutral colors and their priority on skin care, the mineral water they drink and the little naps that keep them looking radiant. Yet in the final analysis, successful French chic boils down to confidence. Without confidence the clothes, neatness, skin care and naps would not translate into French chic.

You can have an American woman who carefully follows the fashion advice of the best fashion magazines and fashion gurus. She follows all the "rules," yet. . . yet, because she is unsure, because she is always looking to others to tell her how she should dress, apply her makeup, and wear her hair, she never quite achieves the stunning personal style she is working to achieve. She never achieves the level of chic that French women do.

CHIC IN ADVERSE SITUATIONS

French chic is the result of thoughtful planning. It requires years of trial and error to achieve perfection anywhere, anytime. When a French woman begins to plan her personal style, she takes into consideration the life she is going to lead. She wants a style that keeps her looking chic in the most adverse situations.

Several years ago, political unrest in Indonesia forced foreign nationals living there to flee. On US news broadcasts, you saw the American business and embassy people at the airport, waiting for planes to evacuate them. These Americans had a harassed, bedraggled, worried look about them.

Then I switched over to the French news on France 2. Here was the report on the French nationals. Most of the French women waiting had short, simple hairstyles. They wore less eyeliner and other makeup than American women. These French women had been sitting in the airport for hours, waiting for a plane, many entertaining small children. They still managed to look chic, attractive, calmly poised. No different than I have seen them waiting for a plane to take a trip back to France for a vacation.

PRIME EXAMPLE OF CHIC

An excellent example of a chic French women's personal style that stood up under the most trying conditions is that of French sailboat racer Isabelle Autissier. When the French woman took the lead in 1999 round the world yacht race, I was so excited I mentioned the achievement on *Chic&Slim* website. The good news soon changed to bad. Isabelle Autissier's sailboat hit a storm and capsized. She spent days in the half-submerged boat until rescued. Along with her rescuers came a news crew. How did she look as she as she was rescued? Neat and chic. The short neat hairstyle looked as if she had just come from a Parisian hairdresser—not from the hull of a sinking boat.

One must experiment to find the right hairstyle that will always work in a lifestyle. But the example of Isabelle Autissier suggests that it is possible no matter what life you lead.

Extremely short hair, the style of which many French women are fond, is not flattering to many of us. I envy women who can wear a short simple haircut, no makeup save a little lip balm and a light brush of blush, and come out looking splendid. Without makeup, I do not look uncomplicated and chic. I look scary.

But after some trial and error (actually, a lot of error), I did come up with a hairstyle that would work well in the humid, windy outdoor life on the South Texas Gulf Coast. My success was testified to by the acquaintance who commented, "You used to have such *wild* hair."

CHIC & CUISINE: THE CONNECTION

To me there has always existed great similarity in the way a French chef approaches the preparation of a French meal and the way a French woman achieves her personal chic. When I read the description of French-born New York chef Pierre Bouley in a *New York Times* review, I was even more convinced. William Grimes wrote that, "As a chef, Bouley has it all—elegance, finesse and flair. His flavors are extraordinarily clear and exquisitely balanced; his use of seasoning is so deft as to be insidious."

The reviewer was impressed that even Bouley's most complex creations had a classical simplicity about them. "Bouley cooks the way Racine wrote and Descartes thought." He continued, "Although French to his fingertips, he has also been traveling, thinking and assimilating foreign influences." This William Grimes believes makes Chef Bouley a more daring chef, and certainly a more exciting one.

In creating their chic, French women also display elegance, finesse, and flair. There is a limpidity and balance to the line of what they wear; French women often dress the way the best of the French writers and thinkers wrote and thought. Chic French women, too, are French from the top of their coiffure to the tips of their high-heeled pumps, yet they often incorporate into their chic influences from other cultures. Quite often their chic has daring that truly makes men see them as exciting and interesting creatures.

CHIC IS FEMININE

Often, it will come up in conversation that I have written a book about French women. So many times, on hearing this, the comment from an American male is, "French women are so feminine." Said a tad wistfully sometimes. But always with great appreciation in the voice. Someone said French women were the epitome of femininity. They probably are. And they enjoy it so!

Not long ago, I received an email from a man who wrote explaining that he was an American who had lived many years in Europe. He said, "I stumbled across your website today and was immediately struck by the profundity of your words." He added, "I have always intuitively felt, but never been able to encapsulate, the essence of European (and French) style. To me, a properly put-together European woman is the most appealing creature on the planet."

Considering that statement, I was not at all surprised to learn that his wife was European.

French women have paid little attention to the women's liberation movement. These women didn't even get the vote until 1946. They like things pretty much as they are, *merci*. These women didn't burn their bras when their sisters in the USA did. These are the women who regularly spend $75 for a bra.

French women's femininity does not mean they never wear jeans or pants. But when they do dress in more traditional masculine clothes, they give their outfits subtle little feminine touches. A young French woman might be wearing a pair of jeans with a long sleeved pullover sweater over a men's tailored Oxford cloth shirt. But you can be sure there will be a pretty ribbon in her hair or dainty earrings, or her grandmother's antique silver bracelet. A French women's magazine featured an article about one of the French women astronauts. Her photograph accompanying the article showed her wearing her flight jacket. Around her neck hung a strand of pearls.

These little feminine French touches aren't only for show. Remember personal style for a French woman is a way of telling the world who she is and what she is about. The ribbon in the hair, like the pearls worn with the flight jacket, are means of expressing a French woman's confidence in and her comfort with her own femininity.

HOW DOES CHIC MAKE SLIM?

Dedicated effort goes into French chic. There are 24 hours in a day. Time and effort devoted to your personal style is time and effort you are *not* devoting to overeating, snacking between meals, being seduced in the supermarket by attractive packaging and displays to buy more food than you need.

In the 1992 movie *Death Becomes Her*, directed by *Forrest Gump* director Robert Zemeckis, Goldie Hawn plays a woman who, when a rival (Meryl Streep) steals her husband (Bruce Willis), she "lets herself go." She gains an enormous amount of weight. The scene of the Goldie Hawn character as fat shows her in an apartment wearing sloppy old sweats, the apartment is dirty and cluttered. Food and empty food containers litter the apartment wall to wall.

Of course, we all know women who are overweight who are meticulous housekeepers. Yet I observe that often very neat, organized women are slim. At the same time, I observe that women whose houses are so littered with accumulated *junque* you would need a team of archeologists to find the kitchen counter top, these women are struggling with excess pounds. (In a later chapter I'll cover in more detail the relationship between household neatness and staying slim.)

Interestingly, I have noticed on various occasions that if I find myself beginning to eat increased quantities of food, or to begin to think up excuses why I might eat a between-meal snack, I'll look around me and find that my living space has become cluttered. If I take a break from the computer and do some straightening, then I am less likely to eat food for which I have no true hunger.

CHIC IS CHOICES

What kind of choices do French women make for their consummate chic maintained with small, well-planned wardrobe?

Esther L. Smith writing in The *Denver Post* said that the number one secret to French chic she learned living in France for five years was that you must pick the piece that defines the season that is right for your age, personality, and lifestyle. Please note that she not only said "defines the season," but also "right for *your* age, personality, and lifestyle." She did not say right for some 17-year-old, six-foot-one anorexic supermodel. (Unless you are, in fact, 17-years-old, six-foot-one, and anorexic.) She wrote, "Basically it's not spending a lot of money that makes French women chic; it's knowing exactly what to buy to suit the season and yourself."

French women show us that chic does not require a lot of clothes, only making the right choices in the few wardrobe additions made each season. How does keeping a small, functional wardrobe affect your weight? For one thing, attitudes in one area of your life often carry over to other areas. When you believe "more is better" when it comes to clothes, it is easy to find yourself stuffing your food pantry as full as you stuff your walk-in closet.

The more food on hand, the more that's available when you get an attack of the munchies.

Also, when you have only a small wardrobe, you don't have all those "fat" clothes hanging there. You know those dresses, pants, and skirts a little on the big side that you wear when you have put on a few pounds. French women have small, perfectly fitting wardrobes. They don't dare gain 100 grams or their clothes won't fit properly. As I wrote in the original *Chic&Slim*, when I began having clothes made by a Parisian-trained dressmaker, the friend who had recommended the woman warned me that the dressmaker made the clothes fit you exactly. I wouldn't be able to gain a pound, or those clothes would not fit properly. She was right. When you have clothes you absolutely love and which make you look wonderful, you don't want to do anything to spoil that wonderful fit and look.

Chic also contributes to slim in yet another way. Finding that those few absolutely right pieces for your wardrobe takes time and diligent effort. And, if you are like French women, searching out really good quality at the best prices, you are going to get a lot of exercise walking the malls and canvassing the dress shops and boutiques.

French women do look for good prices. As authors Dominique Brabec and Égle Salvy write in their book *Paris Chic: The Parisian's Own Insider Shopping Guide:* "Nothing is more chic than buying a bargain or dressing yourself from top to toe in goods with designer labels at knockdown prices. All the Parisians are at it: rummaging around in warehouses, discount stores and bargain basements and still managing to look a million dollars for next-to-nothing!"

While chic plays its vital role in staying slim, what you eat is also important. The French way of eating that keeps them slim and healthy happily breaks many American rules for losing weight and staying slim. The next chapter tells you how the French eat so well and stay so slim.

4

La Cuisine

IF THERE IS ANYTHING AMERICANS ENJOY MORE
than good, rich food, it is the puritanical notion that they should
feel guilty about enjoying good, rich food.

The French do not feel guilty about enjoying good, rich food. Actually,
the French do not feel guilty about enjoying much of anything. Guilt
would put a real drag on that French *joie de vivre*. I often suspect that
in the United States guilt, as much as the caloric and fat content of rich
food, puts the fat on Americans. When I enjoy good, rich food, I do
not feel guilty. Though when I overeat, I sometimes suffer indigestion.

Friends invited me to an elaborate dinner of many courses. Dessert
gave a virtuous performance for the meal's grand finale: a rich cheesecake
blanketed in fresh strawberries marinated in ouzo (that wicked Greek
aperitif). The tipsy berries were then crowned with mascarpone sauce.
Calorie and fat gram count? You wouldn't want to know.

I should have eaten two, perhaps, three small bites of the generous
serving handed me. But intoxicated by the delicious taste (no doubt
with help from the ouzo), my common sense was as inebriated as the
strawberries.

Instead of two or three bites, I ate the serving. The result: I was sick
the entire night.

A few weeks after the ouzo strawberry mascarpone dessert debacle, at a luncheon at the home of another friend, again I was confronted with an American powerhouse dessert. The virtuoso performance grand finale to this meal was also cheesecake. This one was composed of equally rich and intoxicating ingredients. No ouzo (thank goodness), but liberal amounts of chocolate and nuts puréed into the rich body of eggs and cheese. Again, a large American-sized serving arrived on my dessert plate.

The memory of my sleep-depriving gastrointestinal misery prompted restraint. I ate a couple of bites, praised my hostess on her culinary success in the creation, and requested permission to take the rest of my serving home. If I remember correctly, I had a tiny portion of this dessert as an adjunct to my pastry with my afternoon tea for the next four days. My digestive system thanked me. I enjoyed the dessert much more because I ate only a tiny amount each time.

By the way, guilt coupled with indigestion inflicts doubled punishment. If you do say yes to a too-large portion of rich food, at least say no-thank-you to the guilt.

FRENCH SKIP THE GUILT

University psychologist Paul Rozin was quoted by Laura Fraser in a *Salon.com* article on French eating saying the reason the French are slimmer than Americans and have lower rates of coronary artery disease is not *what* they eat, but *how* they eat. (Precisely my point in the original *Chic&Slim*.)

Paul Rozin stresses French positive attitudes toward food. "Talk to a French woman about whether she ever feels guilty about what she eats and she will tell you, as one impossibly young-looking 46-year-old dancer told me, 'Absolutely not—I eat exactly what I please.'"

The good old puritanical guilt Americans know so well is missing from the French mentality. Does the lack of such feelings when enjoying rich food explain why the French can eat all those egg-rich sauces, high-fat cheeses, and superfatted pâtés with so little ill effect to their svelte, oh-la-la French bodies?

A friend returning from a two-week visit in France commented: "Surviving France requires strenuous effort. You spend hours studying your options—most of which are written on menus." True.

No country in the world offers such diversity of good, well-prepared food as France. I can think of no other nation in the world in which the citizens as a whole so revere good, well-prepared food. So with all this eating, all this focus on food, simple lack of puritanical guilt cannot explain why the French can eat so well and stay so slim. Nor can it explain why Americans can spend millions on low-fat and diet foods and see obesity statistics continually rise. Other factors are at work here. This chapter sets out to define for you those specific attitudes, practices, and foods that enable the French to eat all that wonderful French cuisine and still stay slim. I also want to make you aware of those too-common American attitudes, practices, and foods that work against good health and a slim figure. After you read this chapter and put some of its techniques into practice, you should be able to eat as well, yet stay as slim, as those chic French women.

THE EUROPEAN WEIGHT-LOSS SYNDROME

"I spent two weeks in Europe. Every day I ate all this wonderful food. And I lost weight." Extraordinary how many people have said these exact words to me. Incredible, isn't it? Americans visiting Europe tell themselves: "Okay, I am only here for such a short time. Forget watching my weight. I'll eat what I want." So they do. They return to the USA, step on the scales and find they have *lost* five pounds.

Allure magazine gave the phenomena a name, calling it "The European Weight-Loss Syndrome" and running a short feature about it a couple of years ago. Invariably, when Americans take themselves out of their low-fat, no-fat, sugarless, convenience food, instant food, diet food culture, and immerse themselves for a week or two in the real, made-from-scratch, higher fat foods our European cousins eat, they lose weight.

Almost inevitably, it seems, when you begin to eat more as the Europeans do, the American fat begins to melt. (It was certainly true for me.) But what about after the visit to Europe is over? Can you make The European Weight-Loss Syndrome work for you when you are not on vacation in Europe? You can. To learn how to do it, first we need to analyze what is different about the *way* the French and Americans eat. Let's start with real food.

REAL FOOD

Despite McDonald's, KFC, and other fast food franchises popping up across the French landscape like *champignons* after a rain, by and large the French are still eating real food, both in more traditional French eating establishments and at home.

Despite excellent restaurants, caterers, delicatessens, and discriminating home cooks who are preparing healthy, delicious dishes from fresh, natural ingredients, by and large Americans are eating a lot of processed pseudo-food.

Real food vs. pseudo-food? Bread is an excellent example. Take the French baguette, that long, slender baton of chewy, crisp-crusted bread consumed three meals a day every day of the year by almost every Frenchman. By law, those French baguettes are flour, water, yeast, and salt. Nothing more. Nothing less. The French take the quality of their daily bread so seriously they have even recently passed a law that the establishment selling the bread may not call itself a *boulangerie* unless all parts of the bread-making process are done on the premises. Only this artisan bread will qualify a French bread store to call itself a *boulangerie*.

Bread for which the flour, water, salt, and yeast has been mixed elsewhere, pre-formed and shipped to the bakery to be baked and sold there is considered industrial bread. An artisan who makes the bread and sells it in his place of business is an *boulanger*. But a person who only bakes and sells the pre-formed industrial breads is a *fabricant de pain industrial*. A maker of industrial bread. His place of business is not a *boulangerie*, but a cooking terminal for industrial bread or bread depot.

"Industrial bread" made with quality flour by artisans not on the premises where baked can be very good bread. Unfortunately, much of it tastes like what you find in American supermarkets labeled French bread. That is, a poor imitation of good French bread.

So what is the difference between industrial and artisan bread if the ingredients are the same, if equal quality of flours is used in both? "Taste," answered Vincent Ferniot, *critique culinaire* for France 2 television network. He said the difference that gives the artisan bread the superior taste is rising time determined by whether bakers use rapid-rise industrial yeast or more traditional baker's yeast. Remember that in your own bread baking.

Artisan bread rises slowly, allowing a natural fermentation to take place. This makes the distinctive holes in the baked bread and also gives its wonderful taste. According to Julia Child, who has probably written the definitive instructions in English on baking French bread, the slow rise is done at around 70 degrees Fahrenheit. That is cooler than the "warm place" Americans usually allow their bread to rise.

France 2 also interviewed an artisan baker who added that "industrial bread does not sing as artisan bread does." Singing is that lovely cracking sound that the crusty loaves make as they are taken from the oven and begin to cool at room temperature. When you go into a French *boulangerie* and hear bread singing, you know it is truly fresh and truly quality bread.

If the restrictions on what a bakery may call itself seem fussy, some French are even willing to pay more to know the location and ecology of the land on which the wheat used in their loaf was cultivated. They want the same information about their loaf of bread as for their bottle of wine that lists the estate where the grapes were grown and the wine made.

On this side of the Atlantic, many Americans never bother to look, and consequently, don't realize that the bread in that plastic bag on the supermarket shelf may have been baked and sliced in a different (and distant) state. You may be able to find breads baked from only that basic quartet of bread ingredients (flour, water, salt, yeast), but more likely the ingredients label on your bread will be similar to the one I listed in the original *Chic&Slim*. That bread provided an excellent example of highly processed, chemical-laden pseudo-foods Americans are increasingly eating. That bread package listed 30 ingredients, including such tasty-sounding ones as calcium peroxide, calcium stearoyl-2-lactylate, ethoxylated mono and diglycerides, ferrous sulfate, monocalcium phosphate, and ammonium sulfate. Although it was supposed to be geared toward those who wanted to control their weight, this bread contained, not one, but two kinds of sugar.

A DIFFERENT BREED OF CHICKEN

Here is another example of a basic food that the American food industry is currently serving up a pseudo version. The label on the can I picked up said Chicken Broth. True, chicken broth was one of the ingredients in the can so labeled. Yet holding number one position on the label doesn't mean much; water is the major ingredient in chicken broth and there is no way to know if this was one chicken (or one chicken neck) boiled up in 2 quarts of water or two gallons. Then there are the other ingredients in the can: salt, chicken fat, monosodium glutamate, sugar, natural flavor, maltrodextrin, autolyzed yeast extract, modified corn starch, caramel color, disodium inosinate, disodium guanylate, beta carotene (for color), partially hydrogenated soybean oil. Did you notice in fifth place, there was sugar again. Why sugar?

Compare the ingredients in that commercial chicken broth to Julia Child's recipe for chicken broth in *The French Chef Cookbook*: chicken, salt, carrots, celery, leeks, onions, and the seasonings cloves, parsley, bay, and thyme, and beef bones. (For the broth's thickening gelatin, in France, they often use a calf's foot. You can make a nice chicken broth without any form of beef, however.)

Why can't the food industry just boil up some chicken parts with some vegetables and spices the way Julia Child and the French do, and put that in a can? I think the answer is that they would not make as much profit. Monosodium glutamate, sugar, maltrodextrin, autolyzed yeast extract, modified corn starch, disodium inosinate, disodium

AN EXAMPLE: OLIVE OIL

Depending on the region in which olives are grown, quality of the olives, processing of the oil, and the age of the oil, olive oil can taste sourly greasy—or it can taste divine—like a food gift from benevolent gods. Yet, whether blah or delicious, a tablespoon (15 ml.) of olive oil has 120 calories. If you are adding olive oil to give flavor, you must use more of a poorer quality olive oil to produce suitable flavor.

The French are insistent on the best quality oils; they know that they will use less high quality oil to achieve the taste they want. Cold-pressed walnut oil is a nut oil of which the French are particularly fond. Good walnut oil is expensive. But it takes such a small amount of good walnut oil to give that gorgeous flavor to your salad.

In restaurants, I have watched some (invariably overweight) person at the salad bar ladling a half cup or more dressing over their salad. Salad is a generous description of the wilted lettuce leaves, half green tomato slices, grated processed cheese, and bacon bits on the plate. The dressing is invariably a commercial one made with partially hydrogenated salad oil and starchy fillers. When I observe someone using such a large amount of commercial salad dressing, I know if someone tried to put the same quantity of a good French vinaigrette made with high-grade olive oil and a tangy red wine vinegar over the same amount of salad, they could not eat it. The flavors would be too strong; it would make a soupy mess on the plate. Trying to fork salad to mouth without dripping oil on the shirt front would be difficult. No wonder the French can happily sprinkle a tiny amount of the oil and vinegar over their salad greens.

While we are on the subject of salads, I must mention the difference it can make to the taste of a salad if you make it with fresh, flavorful lettuces, wild as well as cultivated. No surprise many Americans don't care much for salad when salad translates to some chopped, tasteless iceberg lettuce combined with slices of equally tasteless supermarket tomatoes (gassed to turn them red, but still unripe) and, tasteless watery, (sometimes bitter) cucumber, leaving it to a poor little slivered green onion to give the salad some taste.

When I have really good, fresh salad lettuce or greens, often I don't even need any oil to provide a satisfying delicious taste. Just a squeeze of fresh lemon juice, a touch of salt, and a bit of freshly ground white or black pepper, and I have a superb salad.

ANOTHER EXAMPLE: SEA SALT

This leads us to the topic of another basic cooking ingredient: salt. Anyone who has ever been prescribed a salt-free or salt-reduced diet knows that without salt, many foods are extremely unappealing. Ordinary American table salt is mined and comes with an added anticaking agent (yellow prussiate of soda—doesn't that sound yummy?) to make certain it pours freely from the shaker even in the most humid weather.

The French prefer to season their food with sea salt. Many proclaim a passionate preference for sea salt evaporated from waters on the Normandy coast. Good sea salt gives a saltier taste with less salt than regular salt. (A definite health and weight control advantage.) Another nutritional advantage is trace minerals in salt evaporated from sea water.

POWERHOUSE FLAVOR FRUITS

The French often eat a piece of fruit with no added sugar instead of a higher-calorie dessert. Many Americans on a diet try to replace their usual pistachio marshmallow cherry ice cream with an apple or an orange. They find the substitution unsatisfactory. To give the sweetness satisfaction of a highly sugared dessert, fresh fruit has to be high quality, sweet and pungent with flavor. Unfortunately so much fruit sitting on the supermarket shelves is bred for large size and appearance rather than flavor. Picked green and shipped some great distance, it arrives at the store more unripe than ripe.

Even when markets in the USA offer quality fruit, many Americans, particularly those of the younger generations who have grown up in the pseudo-food age, don't know how to choose quality fruit. In the produce section of my supermarket, I encountered a young woman I knew. Both she and her husband were overweight, she probably 100 pounds. He was of a size, combined with his inactive lifestyle and fried food diet, gave him good odds of a heart attack around age 42.

She said she was buying bananas for her husband. She chose a bunch, every banana as green as a tree leaf. "When does he intend to eat them?" I asked. They would probably be edible in two weeks to a month. "When I get home," she answered, puzzled by my question. "They're green," I pointed out somewhat redundantly. "He likes them this way," she said.

As they were: starchy, bitter, hard, with none of the custard sweetness and creamy texture of a properly ripe banana, there was little chance that a banana from that bunch would provide the dessert satisfaction of cake or cookies. So husband would eat the fruit without much enjoyment, perhaps because he thought he should eat fruit for health, then he would hit the bag of chocolate chip chewies or the oatmeal raisin bars for something that satisfied his desire for sweet.

Just for the record, bananas are not at their proper ripeness for eating until they are well freckled. Buy them yellow a few days before you plan to eat them. Bring them home and put them in a fruit bowl. Never refrigerate a banana. Let them ripen at room temperature until well freckled. If you cannot eat a banana at its peak ripeness, peel, slice, put it in a freezer container or plastic bag and freeze it. Later, put frozen banana slices in a blender with about 1/4 cup skim milk, soy milk, or rice milk. Process until milk shake texture. This banana whip will satisfy ice cream or frozen yogurt cravings. You can add a bit of sugar, honey, or other sweetener, if you think the flavor requires it. But if the bananas are truly ripe (and you have been lucky enough to buy a reasonably good banana), and if your sweetness expectation level is more that of chic French women rather than that of the average American, no additional sweetening will be needed.

BREAKFAST CEREAL IS NOT CHIC

How did it happen? How did the United States go from a culture of immigrants who brought with them established traditions of bread baking to a culture that abandoned crusty, flavorful bread for some flavorless, processed breakfast flakes? The story is as edifying as it is horrifying. A textbook case of how Nouveaux Puritans with good marketing techniques can do a great deal of harm while meaning to do a great deal of good. That story can be read other places. (For example, in T. Coraghessan Boyle's novel *The Road to Wellville,* or in a biography of Dr. John Harvey Kellogg.) Suffice to say here that another major difference in the way the French eat, and the way Americans eat, is choice of breakfast foods. Many Americans breakfast on dry, cold commercial cereal. When I was a fatty, I ate ready-to-eat cereal, a "low-calorie," supposedly nutritious one created for dieters. I ate it with skim milk and artificial sweetener. Only when I replaced my American diet cereal breakfast with a traditional French breakfast did I successfully lose weight and stay slim.

The traditional French breakfast is coffee or tea and a small roll with butter and jam. Or, instead of the roll, a chunk of good French baguette. The French call this preparation a *tartine,* meaning something that has been spread. Bread used in a *tartine* is, of course, that good French bread made without added fats, sugar, and chemicals. If you have ever watched a chic French women spread butter on her *tartine,* you know she takes this very small amount of butter and then spreads, and spreads, and spreads. This process takes so long that I have always suspected they burn up more calories spreading the butter than are actually in the butter. The French insist on the richest, creamiest, freshest butter. So a very small amount gives a lovely butter taste. (Another example of how you need less of a quality product.)

As for the jam, the French like to make (or purchase) jams from fruit sweetened with natural fruit juice. In most American jams, at least on the labels I find on my supermarket shelf, the principal ingredient these days seems to be high fructose corn syrup. Fruit often comes in second place. Unfortunately, sugar often comes in third. High fructose corn syrup (a form of refined sugar) plus refined sugar equals lots of sugar and not much fruit.

Then there is pectin to make up for the fact that there's not much fruit. When spreading jam or jelly on their breakfast bread, Americans are basically spreading sugar with a bit of fruit for flavoring. When spreading jam or jelly on their breakfast *tartine,* the French are basically

nutritional authorities define a standard serving size of meat as three and one-half to four ounces. Once, in an American restaurant, I was seated next to a man of great appetite and great girth. His steak arrived, a thick eight-ounce slab. I must have looked shocked. "That's an average serving," he said defensively. "Twelve or sixteen ounces would be a large serving."

Or you could eat the whole cow, I thought. But I said, "I believe that an average serving is currently defined as three and a half to four ounces." Who had defined it? I couldn't remember. The US Department of Agriculture or the American Heart Association possibly. He scoffed. Like many Americans, he believed it was his God-given and Constitutional right to overeat.

Whether or not we have divine or legal right to overeat red meat, or any other food, the latest medical research indicates that overeating is taking a serious toll on our health. In the traditional American resistance to moderation, as soon as these research findings were published, media articles appeared asking if overeating curtailed one's life, might not starving yourself prolong it?

William R. Clark, University of California Los Angeles professor emeritus of immunology and author of *A Means to an End: The Biological Basis of Aging and Death*, concluded that what the full body of research suggests is: excess caloric intake shortens maximal life span, but caloric restriction does not extend it. Overeating can shorten your life. But starving yourself will not make you live longer. We know why. Overeating leads to excess weight. Excess weight is related directly and indirectly to many health problems.

What research by Professor Clark and others tells us is that the French habit of moderate portions of a variety of healthy, natural foods seems to be the best ticket toward living a long, healthy life. Peter Mayle has written charmingly on the French lifestyle and eating habits. In his 1999 book *Encore Provence,* he commented on the French practices of eating at meals rather than snacks and on drinking red wine with meals:

...I have a feeling that there are other less dramatic influences at work on and in the French stomach. I believe, without a shred of scientific proof, that the raw ingredients (in France) contain fewer additives, preservatives, colorants, and chemical novelties than in the States. I also believe that food eaten at a table is better for you than food eaten hunched over a desk, standing at a counter, or driving in a car. And I believe that, wherever you do it, hurried eating has ruined more digestive systems than foie gras.

SMOKING

Why are the French satisfied with a moderate portion size? Some Americans insist it is because the French smoke. What about smoking? What role does it play in weight control for French women? Why is smoking not even mentioned in the original *Chic&Slim*?

Americans often try to credit French slimness to smoking. But look at the facts. An article in the December 1999 *Self* magazine titled "Stay Slim Secrets of Women Who Eat What They Want: Self Goes to Paris to Learn How The Western World's Thinnest Women Get Away With Eating And Drinking As They Please", points out that 27 percent of French women smoke and 24 percent of American women smoke. That is only 3 percent difference. Not much. Yet, depending on whose figures you use, 33 percent to more than 50 percent of all American women are overweight. Also, if 27 percent of French women smoke, that still leaves 73 percent of French women who do *not* smoke. Yet only 6 to 8 percent of French women are overweight. That means that the majority of French women are *not* overweight. The majority of French women do *not* smoke.

We all know overweight women who smoke. Smoking is no guarantee of slimness, though smoking is said to jazz up the metabolism and make you burn calories more rapidly. Regular exercise will do the same thing—but without the negative side effects. Smoking is said to suppress the appetite. But some French women claim that it is really that high-octane French coffee that suppresses their appetite (as well as supercharges them for energy through a busy day). Satisfying the appetite with good healthy food rather than refined sugar snacks also keeps the appetite regulated. Active lifestyles also play a role.

The reasons I did not mention smoking in the original *Chic&Slim* was principally because the book's purpose was to share those lessons that I had learned from French women about how they lose weight and stay slim, those lessons that I had incorporated into my own system. Smoking certainly is *not* part of the *Chic&Slim* system. Also, a great many of the French women from whom I learned important lessons in weight control did not smoke. In fact, they were extremely opposed to smoking. They thought it was terrible for the skin, for one thing. And quite frankly, a number of the French women I knew simply could not afford to smoke. Still, they were chic and slim.

Puritanical Americans love to say that the French are slim because they smoke. This way these Americans avoid admitting other things that the French are doing right, the things covered in *Chic&Slim*, such as eating in moderation, small portions, avoiding junk food snacks, and living active lives.

Women's health authority Dr. Susan Love, writes in *The Hormone Book*: "There's no question that smoking is the single most dangerous thing you can do in terms of your overall health. It causes premature menopause (and wrinkles)—and that's the least of it." According to Dr. Love, smoking increases the risk of heart disease, osteoporosis, and certain cancers.

Dr. Love also points out that studies have shown that the most common reason women give for not quitting smoking is their fear of gaining weight. She recommends that you develop other methods of losing weight and reducing stress—such as exercise—before you try to quit smoking.

I agree with Dr. Love that you should begin lifestyle changes that will help you lose weight and deal with stress *before* you try to give up your cigarette habit. After you have incorporated some of the *Chic&Slim* changes into your lifestyle, you may decide that your cigarette breath and clothes reeking of tobacco smoke may not be a part of your chic personal style. That personal style decision might be the incentive you need to give up smoking. Learning to live and eat *Chic&Slim* will surely keep you from gaining weight when you do give up smoking.

MY FRIEND FAT

When they write the history of weight loss in the second half of the 20th century, under the heading of "Things That In Hindsight Were Not Such a Good Idea" will be low-fat.

Not that it isn't a good idea to use moderation in eating fried foods, red meats, cheeses, chips, and pastries rich in butter. But that wasn't the remedy employed. When medical experts announced that Americans were eating a diet too high in fats for people who lead increasingly inactive lifestyles, the United States food industry seized that opportunity to create and market a whole array of "low-fat" versions of many foods. In many, simple starches and sugars replaced the fat in the original version. Any number of confusions and problems ensued.

Likely more from wishful thinking than careful reading of labels, many individuals translated the words "low-fat" on the package into "non-fat." More troublesome still, many translated "low-fat" as "low-calorie." They began eating low-fat sandwich meat or low-fat cookies as if they were some extremely low-calorie vegetables such as lettuce, alfalfa sprouts, or green beans.

Low-fat created gurus. Interestingly, two who achieved popularity originated their programs in Texas, a state not known for traditional low-fat cuisine. Best-loved Texas foods such as steaks (inevitably served with an enormous baked potato dripping butter or sour cream), barbecue, chili, and enchiladas are all on the high end of the fat-in-food scale. Favorite desserts like pecan pie topped with a big dollop of ice cream are not *on* the high end of the fat-in-food scale; they *are* the high end. No surprise that both these Texas-originating gurus, at the time of this writing, are headquartered in more low-fat friendly locales on the West Coast: Los Angeles and Seattle.

Dr. Dean Ornish's program is medically oriented and geared toward individuals hoping to heal or prevent serious heart disease. The other

Texas-originating guru focuses on exercise and fitness. Remember Susan Powter? She, the abrasive Dallas exercise studio owner with her supershort haircut and her rage, screaming: "IT'S FAT THAT MAKES YOU FAT!"

Susan's system made it simple. You *never* ate any food with more than 28 percent fat. That eliminated a great many French favorites: Camembert, foie gras, *bifstek, brioche, saucisson, croissants au beurre*. . .

Susan Powter acquired a large following after the publication of her first book, *Stop The Insanity*. She generated much media coverage, partly because of her unique personal style: bleached hair about one-quarter inch long all over her head, her face most usually contorted by rage, and a voice screaming in anger.

The best article on Susan Powter I read was in *Texas Monthly* magazine written by Jan Jarboe. While working on the article, Jan Jarboe subjected herself to the Powter regime for six (not very happy) weeks. Her conclusion: "I'd lost fifteen pounds. Yet I was mad at the whole damn world, just like Powter. Eating a steady stream of bagels, beans, and baked potatoes had been a mood-altering experience. The entire time I was on the diet I was cranky, ready to do battle with anyone who got in my way."

Low-fat, however, was merely the subtext to Susan Powter's weight-loss message. The overriding message was anger: anger at men, at the "diet" industry, at the aerobics industry, at lawyers, and at beauty product manufacturers. Most of all, the low-fat guru was angry at men. Susan Powter told women, "Stop trying to live up to the expectations of the men in your life since you get neither appreciation nor help with the housework in return."

Susan Powter's message had little chance becoming popular in France. French women believe it well worth the effort to try and please men. In return, French men give appreciation for French women's efforts—though their appreciation takes other forms than helping with housework. French men help even less around the house than American men. French women deal with that matter simply by arranging their households for minimal housework that they take care of themselves. (More about that in the next chapter.)

BACKLASH

Not long after Susan Powter's diet guru popularity peaked, the diet pendulum made a giant swing away from low-fat. Should we have been surprised? No. Inevitably, denial is followed by backlash. In the case of low-fat, for many, it had been almost 30 years of denial. Americans, fed up with the flavorless, often more expensive than the real, low-fat pseudo-foods the food industry packaged up for them, discarded low-fat. They embraced new gurus. New high-fat, high-protein gurus proclaimed you could eat all the steak, fried eggs, barbecued ribs, lobster in butter you wanted. The catch? You had to avoid carbohydrates. You could have bacon and fried eggs for breakfast, but you couldn't have any toast and jam to go with them. You could have your steak, but not your baked potato. Pies and other desserts remained forbidden.

One of the gurus, Dr. Robert C. Atkins, M.D., was (again) selling zillions of books. I knew one woman on his program, who, for months, ate nary a vegetable, nor slice of bread. Just all those big fatty steaks, shrimp, lots of chicken and pork. Did she lose weight? Well, actually, no. And I don't think she nor her doctor were happy about the highs her cholesterol levels achieved either.

Both low-fat and high-fat (with ultra-low carbohydrate) programs appealed enormously to Americans who consistently demonstrate what I sometimes believe may be a genetic aversion to moderation, especially when it comes to moderation in food consumption. Both the Ornish and Powter programs could point to adherents' successes. Yet both low-fat programs failed to put a dent in the rapidly rising USA obesity statistics. Americans keep getting fatter and fatter as do the bank accounts of the gurus offering the extreme programs.

For a detailed explanation of the whole "low-fat" phenomena and why we saw an increase in the percentage of the population who became, or remained, overweight while consistently replacing the traditional version of the food with "low-fat," you can read *Low Fat Lies: High*

Fat Frauds and the Healthiest Diet in the World. The book's authors, Dr. Mary Flynn, a nutritionist, and Dr. Kevin Vigilante, a medical professor, are both affiliated with Brown University. Their message was that not only were low-fat diets boring, unpalatable, and often left you hungry, they were also potentially dangerous. They could lower your good cholesterol and raise harmful triglycerides. They might also hinder absorption of carotenes that combat cancer, heart disease and other diseases. What they recommended as they best way to health and normal weight was the "Mediterranean" way of eating. This, of course, is the style of eating of southern France. It was, incidentally, the type of eating done by the French woman Jeanne Calment, who achieved such a stunning age of 122 despite a lifelong cigarette habit.

Drs. Flynn and Vigilante are not the only ones pointing out the problems with the low-fat and high-fat diet crazes. Dr. Alice H. Lichtenstein, a professor of nutrition at Tufts University in Boston, was quoted in a 1999 *New York Times* article saying: "People assumed that if a food had no fat, they could eat as much of it as they wanted. But many low-fat and fat-free products have nearly as many calories as their full-fat versions."

Too many people believed that cutting back on fat alone would guarantee weight loss. They missed the point that you have to cut calories or increase physical activity. Dr. Lichtenstein recommended fat at 30 percent of calories in the American daily food quota. True, Mediterranean diets often had as much as 40 percent fat, but she said: "If we go above that (30 percent), Americans tend to increase their consumption of saturated fats in meats. Maybe if we adopted a Mediterranean diet—rich in vegetables and fish and olive oil—we could go higher than 30 percent fat without compromising our health." Dr. Lichtenstein went on to point out that the Mediterraneans' low rate of heart disease wasn't just the result of their diet. These people lead a more active lifestyle than that generally followed in the USA. They don't eat all the "bizarre" foods Americans do.

American supermarkets shelves do offer an extraordinary number of bizarre pseudo-foods. Most I manage to ignore. But every once in a while, some supermarket employee presses a sample upon me. All these pseudo-food samples I have been offered impress me with the creativity that has gone into creating an appealing package. I understand that today the food industry often first creates an attractive package, then, it comes up with a product to sell inside the package. Marketing gimmicks of these pseudo-foods are invariably clever. Often, they appeal to a sense of nostalgia. Or they make claims about health. Often debatable claims. Ingredients invariably turn out to be some combination of sugar, flour, partially hydrogenated oil, flavoring (usually artificial) and chemicals whose names seem to consist of two words of at least five syllables.

As for nostalgia, if you want something that tastes "as good as Grandma's," you should assemble butter, flour, a little sugar, and some cinnamon and make cookies.

For a while, I would taste supermarket pseudo-food samples out of curiosity. After several left an unpleasant taste in my mouth, and a couple upset my stomach, I now no-thank-you them. I tried feeding sample crackers to the omnivorous seagulls that hung around the beach behind my Corpus Christi condo. But the seagulls spit out the crackers and refused to eat them. I guess that should tell us something.

Americans see fat in food as bad. They continually invent pseudo-foods that have eliminated all or a great deal of the fat normally present in the real version. Many of these low-fat pseudo-foods would surely qualify as the bizarre foods to which Dr. Lichtenstein refers.

But the French know that a moderate amount of fat can help you lose weight, or maintain your normal weight. For one thing, fat in food makes it taste good. A ratatouille, the Provençale vegetable casserole made of onions, tomatoes, eggplant, zucchini, and garlic, makes a good example. Without olive oil, these cooked vegetables are just that, a dish of cooked vegetables. But flavor them with a rich, high-quality virgin olive oil, roast them slowly in moderate heat, and the casserole takes on such a meaty flavor that it will replace a meat dish of a much higher number of calories. You won't feel hungry two hours after eating as you might if you ate only plain low-cal vegetables. Fat keeps you feeling full.

The French are realists. They know that a few calories of a quality fat such as butter, walnut oil, or olive oil, or the flavorful fat cooked from natural meats, or almond paste in an elegant dessert can make foods taste sufficiently good you will be more inclined to eat a balanced diet of vegetables, whole grains, and proteins.

NON-FAT. NON!

It was from the French that I learned to eat yogurt. Before I discovered yogurt at the *crémerie* in little plastic tubs, I can't remember tasting it. By the early 1970s, yogurt was available in American supermarkets, as well as in health food stores. Many American supermarket brands contained pectin and food starch and other additives I preferred not to have in my yogurt. I begin making my own. The quart jar of milk and starter in a warm place method did not prove altogether satisfactory. When I saw a yogurt maker advertised for sale, I bought. That counter top appliance, a warming tray with five inset individual containers, by the way, is still making wonderful yogurt.

Not long after I embarked on my homegrown yogurt making, the subject of this healthy, cultivated dairy product came up at a dinner party. I mentioned my new yogurt maker. A French woman with whom I was chatting said that she too made her own yogurt. We agreed on the advantages of homemade yogurt: better taste, more economical, no additives such as were often added to commercial brands of yogurt. "And low-fat." I said.

"*Non!*" she said firmly. "You must make yogurt from whole milk."

"But the calories, the fat," I protested.

"*Non.*" She repeated that firm French negative that discourages argument. "The taste of whole milk yogurt is so much better." And that was the end of that discussion.

I looked at the French woman. Not an ounce overweight. Perfect skin, glowing with health, beautiful, shiny hair. She ate whole milk yogurt because it tasted better. And it does. A good brand of whole fat yogurt can taste like a *crème fraîche*. And did you ever calculate how many calories you were saving eating that less tasty non-fat yogurt? Less than four calories per tablespoon. Three and three-quarters of a calorie, actually.

When you are using yogurt as a substitute for sour cream in a dip or as topping for a baked potato, the difference in taste is usually worth those few calories difference. At least, chic French women think so.

FEAR OF FOOD

Many American women today appear actually afraid of food. Of course, French women do not fear food. The chief emotions that food provokes in French women are pleasure and satisfaction. How did it come about that some American women began to see good, well-prepared food as something bad to avoid? When I left the USA in the mid-1960s, good food was still held in high regard. But especially in the 1980s and 1990s, you actually saw women restrict themselves to the harshest of regimens, shunning all foods that one normally thinks of as enjoyable.

Perhaps the idea of enjoyable foods as "bad" had something to do with the nomenclature chosen by one of the major weight control programs for the foods allowed on their diet and those not allowed: legal and illegal. It was during these same years that the drug culture blossomed in the USA. We became aware of two kinds of drugs. There was the high blood pressure medicine your grandmother took, which was legal. And there was marijuana, LSD, cocaine, which were illegal. The illegal drugs could have some unwanted side effects. Landing you in jail was one of them. Death by drug overdose was another. So the thinking went that illegal foods were those that were bad for you.

Women began to fear food and began eating only low-cal veggies with some low-fat protein. Their bodies thought it was famine time. Their metabolisms dutifully slowed down. Their bodies reached a state in which they truly could *not* eat more than a very low-calorie restricted diet or they would gain weight.

Paul Rozin at the University of Pennsylvania has done studies on food attitudes on the part of the Americans and French. He found that Americans have greater concerns about what they eat and are much more dissatisfied with what they eat than the French. That stress leads Americans to poor eating habits, extreme dieting, bingeing, overeating, and obsessing about food. All of which are unhealthy.

Laura Fraser writes in *Salon.com*, "The real paradox, Rozin says, isn't that the French enjoy food and remain thin and heart disease-free. It's that Americans worry so much about food, do so much more to control their weight and end up so much more dissatisfied with their meals."

Need I say it? Americans end up so much more overweight.

BRILLAT-SAVARIN ENCORE

If French women have no fear of food, perhaps this comes from taking to heart the pronouncements of Brillat-Savarin. Jean-Anthelme Brillat-Savarin was the 18th century Frenchman who penned the classic *The Physiology of Taste or Meditations on Transcendental Gastronomy*. It was he who gave us that famous phrase:

You are what you eat.

Monsieur Brillat-Savarin also had theories about women and food. The English translations here are those of American food writer M.F.K. Fisher whose rendering of this famous work from French into English is probably the definitive one.

Brillat-Savarin wrote: "The leanings of the fair sex toward gourmandism are in a way instinctive, for it is basically favorable to their beauty." He went on to say that "…a tempting diet, dainty and well prepared, holds off for a long time the exterior signs of old age." He added that "It adds brilliancy to the eyes, freshness to the skin, and more firmness to all the muscles; and just as it is certain, in physiology, that it is the sagging of these muscles which cause wrinkles, beauty's fiercest enemy, so it is equally correct to say that, other things being equal, the ladies who know how to eat are comparatively ten years younger than those to whom this science is a stranger."

Reading Brillat-Savarin's words, one cannot help but think of Italian actress Sophia Loren, who translated her love of pasta into such a voluptuous figure that, at age 65, in a poll, she was named the "most beautiful woman in the world."

Note that Brillat-Savarin said, "ladies who know how to eat," My goal in writing this book to show you "how to eat well" so that you can enjoy good, well prepared food, yet stay slim and youthful-looking, just as French women do. As Sophia Loren does. In *People* in September 1999, as the actress approached her sixty-fifth birthday an article described Sophia Loren's usual food regimen. I was struck by how closely it parallels this style of eating that I learned from French women and which I am now passing on to you in the *Chic&Slim* books and website.

COOKING FROM SCRATCH

Instant. Convenient. Quick. In the USA, these are favorite food words. Americans are always in a hurry. Too much in a hurry to go through the rigmarole of peeling and chopping fresh vegetables, actually cooking raw meat, measuring ingredients, stirring them together, and then placing in an oven or cooking pan.

Americans adore the mix, the frozen, the pre-prepared, the dehydrated, and the canned. Something else comes into play here, I believe. Advertising has convinced American cooks that they are somehow incompetent to prepare something by themselves. I think of a friend who is a wonderful cook. Yet when she wants to make curry, she buys a curry mix in which to prepare her shrimp or chicken.

I lived two years in India, and I ate a lot of curry, watched a lot of curry prepared, and have continued to make curry in the decades since I left India. Curry requires putting some oil in a pan, adding a little onion and then some curry spices then adding the chicken, shrimp, or whatever you are currying.

If my friend would have a little confidence in her abilities, she could save money using curry powder in her curry instead of the expensive curry mix which, of course, also contains sugar and filler and chemicals that a curry powder does not have. She might even, reach in her spice cabinet, take out cumin, coriander, some mustard and turmeric, and a few other spices and mix up her own curry powder to suit her own preference. (See the recipe section of this book for my curry powder recipe.)

American advertising has convinced Americans that homemade is inferior, when, in almost every comparison with a mix, homemade is superior. Homemade is also generally free from additives and fillers that contribute to ill health and fat.

Americans worry about doing things "right." Chic French women define "right" as the way *they* do something. If you have confidence, you believe in your own ability to prepare food the way you and your family like to eat it.

True, the French now have more frozen foods and mixes than they did three decades ago. But to a far greater extent than in the USA, the French are still preparing three meals a day, cooking from scratch. This habit helps them stay slim. These cooked-from-scratch meals are more palatable, offer more nutrition, and keep the French inclined to eat at meals rather than graze on high-calorie, high-sugar, high-fat snack foods between meals.

I invariably found that dishes these French products produced were of a higher quality than what one would produce from an instant food or mix available in the USA. For instance: powdered milk. Like almost anyone who dieted in the USA in the 1950s and 1960s, I was familiar with "instant non-fat dry milk." A staple of many diet programs, when reconstituted with water to make one cup, it provided a good dose of protein and calcium at only 80 calories. It (then) cost a fraction of fresh milk. You could buy it packaged in one cup foil packets that easily tucked into suitcase or handbag.

On the downside, the taste of instant non-fat dry milk little resembled pasteurized, homogenized milk from a grocery waxed paper carton. Ah, but the *lait écrémé en poudre* sold in French stores was an entirely different matter. True, butterfat and water had been removed, but good milk taste remained when reconstituted. When I read later that the French drank much more skimmed (*écrémé*) milk than Americans, I understood why.

PLATTERS

One French meal custom I found useful for weight control was the habit of serving the food on platters. When presented food on a platter, you were free to help yourself to the portion size that you chose to eat. By the way, most French consider it bad manners to take something on your plate and not finish it. Wasteful. The French do not waste. They especially abhor waste of well-prepared food. Well-prepared food is an art. The food served at a French table is invariably good. If you owned a Picasso, would you hang it facing the wall so you couldn't see it?

In a French home, if the host or hostess was serving my plate, my request for a small size portion would be honored. At French tables I never ran into the problem I so often experience in the USA. I request a small portion and plopped down in front of me is an amount two to three times what I requested. Perhaps some hosts believe that I am only being polite asking for a small amount. In most cases, I am convinced it is simply food pushing. A power thing. Food pushers will try to force me to eat more than I want in order to demonstrate they can make me do something against my wishes. Other times when you encounter this overfilling of your plate in a home, it is a competitive effort to keep you from losing weight or to cause you to gain weight. Please be a considerate host or hostess. When a guest requests a small serving, do them the courtesy of honoring their request. If they say no thank you, show them the respect of acknowledging that they know what is best for their own health.

MEAL TIME CONVERSATION

French requirements for a good meal: good food, good wine, good conversation, good company. If you have the latter, good company, then you are more likely to have the next-to-latter requirement: good conversation. Many of us were raised in families in which certain topics were acceptable for table conversation, others not. Unfortunately, in the USA, mealtimes are no longer the civilized affairs they once were. Table conversation can have an effect on your weight.

We know that food eaten slowly when people are relaxed digests better; chances increase that food will be well metabolized becoming fuel, not stored fat. When food is eaten slowly in a relaxed atmosphere, more often you are satisfied with a smaller amount of food.

The French still moderate mealtime conversation with standards of civility. Certain topics are not discussed. One cultivates the art of making pleasant conversation that will not bore, yet at the same time not disturb anyone's digestion.

THE ART OF LIVING (AND EATING) CONSCIOUSLY

In the original *Chic&Slim* and elsewhere, I have written that much American overeating is done mindlessly. The overeater is oblivious to gobbling down food while watching television, driving a car, walking down the street, or talking on the phone. The French concentrate on their food at designated mealtimes. This prevents mindless overeating, as well as promotes better digestion.

Psychologist Dr. Nathaniel Branden's book T*he Art of Living Consciously* deals with problems people cause themselves when they do things without giving them their full attention. He also provides techniques whereby one can improve all areas of one's life by living in a more conscious manner.

Living consciously, in its most basic definition, seems to be: paying attention and having your mind focused on what you are doing at the time you are doing it. One way the French derive pleasure from life, and stay slim in the process, is their habit of doing things in a very conscious, deliberate matter with their minds focused on the matter at hand. This is true whether they are shopping for fresh produce, in conversation with another person, making love, or eating a meal.

AROMA

One thing the more leisurely French approach to eating allows is the opportunity to enjoy the aroma of the food as well as the taste.

The Frenchman invariably fills his wine glass not to the top, but only about two-thirds full. He knows the bulbous shape of the wine glass will allow the bouquet to form in the air in the empty upper portion of the glass and be held there. When the glass is raised to the nose, the wine's bouquet will delight him even before the wine itself has touched his tongue. Wine offers two pleasures: the first to the nose, the second to the palate.

I remember French dinners in which the dish—my memories are particularly vivid for fish baked in a wonderful sauce—was brought to the table on a covered platter. At tableside, the server would raise the lid with a flourish allowing the fragrant aroma to rise up in a cloud and hover over us like some friendly culinary spirit. Many good restaurants bring the food to the table covered. This not only ensures that the food will arrive at the table at a temperature that best allows you to enjoy it, but the cover also holds the aroma ready to please you at the table. Aroma serves as a kind of prelude to the symphony of flavor in the dish itself.

The French derive pleasure from their food because they take the time to enjoy the wonderful aromas of food and beverages. If you take time to enjoy the aroma of the food you are eating, not only will the aroma enhance the taste and increase your pleasure, but taking the time to enjoy the aroma is useful to slow your pace of eating.

Americans always look for a silver bullet: They say that it is the red wine that keeps the French slim and healthy. Or it is the olive oil and fish. Or eating meals in courses. In actual fact, as I have tried to show you in this chapter, it is the *way* food is prepared and eaten as well as *food choices* that add up to eating pleasure and to slim, healthy bodies.

The way French women organize their households also helps keep them chic and slim.

5

LE SHOPPING & LA DÉCO

THE POOR FRENCH! HOW I PITIED THEM WHEN I SAW their homes. Compared to people in the United States, they didn't have much stuff. As for shopping, they were truly disadvantaged. Stores lacked shopping carts. Customers had to provide their own shopping bags to carry home their purchases.

When I first began observing French culture several decades ago, I was still firmly of the American mentality that believed quality of life was directly connected to how many material possessions one had. The preparation of good food, to my American way of thinking, was directly related to a modern kitchen equipped with electric mixers, spacious refrigerators with generous freezer compartments, kitchen ranges with four burners, an oven that would accommodate a large Thanksgiving turkey sufficient for scores of relatives, and a broiler that could handle six 12-ounce steaks with room to spare. To supply this modern equipment required cabinets filled with convenience products. The good life also required shopping centers with large supermarkets and larger parking lots.

Yet the French, poor souls! Trudging from the *crémerie* to the *boulangerie* to the *charcutier* to the *marchand de viande* to the *marchand de poisson* to the *épicerie*. Butter and eggs one place, bread and pastries in another. Pork and sausages in one shop, beef in another, fish in yet another. Flour, spices, and your box of Omo laundry detergent sold down the street.

Those first French homes I visited looked bare in comparison to American homes. Bathrooms lacked those decorator items with which Americans cozy up that room of the house. Monastic is a word often used (appropriately) for French bedrooms. A French bedroom might be only large enough for the bed and a small bedside table, perhaps one chair.

Initially, I pitied the French with their shopping inconveniences and their minimalist decorated homes. In time, I learned that possessing fewer consumer goods did not diminish the French quality of life. In fact, having less "stuff" contributed to the French enjoyment of life. Furthermore, the uncluttered French households and the French system of shopping on a daily, or almost daily, basis played a vital role in keeping French women chic and slim.

Better still, I discovered I could use French women's shopping and household arrangement lessons to help me lose weight and stay slim.

SHOPPING DIFFERENCES

Even today, with *supermarchés* and *hypermarchés* common in France, the shopping experience in the two countries is still as different as Paris and Pottawattamie County. At the most basic, merchants in the USA go to great effort and expense to make shopping convenient, pleasant, even fun. In my neighborhood supermarket, they serenade me with music, provide me with maps to help me find products, recipes with which to cook them, special informational displays, flyers listing specials, and coupons for savings. In addition to food, I can buy almost any basic household plumbing, electrical, garden, office, school, or pool supply I might need. While I am shopping for food, I can also buy my auto tags, postage stamps, or a hunting and fishing license. I can cash checks, process photos, eat in their restaurant, wire money, check my blood pressure, have my prescriptions filled, and ship packages. Should I sprain my ankle, they have motorized shopping carts to ferry me around the store.

In France, even when French stores model themselves on American stores, shopping lacks the organized ease and convenience of the USA. For instance, in French food shops, there is always the chance that, if you don't shop early, what you wanted to buy may be sold out.

In French supermarkets, you unload your purchases onto the counter, then, you rush to bag them yourself and tote them to your vehicle, or to public transport, or all the way home on foot or cycle. For most French, I am assured, the *supermarchés* are an ordeal, not a pleasure. In some of the smaller shops where one is an established customer, however, shopping can be more pleasant.

If you have experienced French shopping first hand, you know the general attitude of French merchants toward customers. One French analyst summed up this attitude as "The Customer: Our Enemy." Any of us who have inadvertently violated one of those numerous unwritten rules of French shopping have found that this analysis is not an exaggeration.

French Shopping (An Example)

Once I went with a visiting American friend to buy a tube of toothpaste in a French *pharmacie*. The American managed to violate one of those unwritten rules that earn hostility in a French shop. He pawed through the display of toothpastes, hoping to find an American brand. Doing so, he messed up the tidily arranged display. Even though I quickly tried to rearrange the packages, the damage had been done.

In the French way of thinking, you should know the brand of toothpaste you use. You should take the top package from the display. If you are unsure which brand to purchase, you should consult with the *pharmacienne*, and she will recommend the proper one for you. You do not do a messy search on your own.

The slight disorder my American friend created infuriated the French *pharmacienne*. Initially she refused to sell the toothpaste. It took my most abject pleas offered in French, before she, still furious, finally snatched the offered money and rang up the sale.

If I had been able to restrain my impetuous American friend, I would have approached the *pharmacienne*, consulted with her on what toothpastes were available, let her tell me there were no American brands for sale (which I knew anyway) and allow her to recommend a French brand that might have the flavoring and other properties desired. Why should it be done this way? Because that is the way the French do things. At least in that particular shop.

SHOPPING AMERICAN STYLE

In the original *Chic & Slim*, I wrote that, though most Americans live only minutes away from well-stocked supermarkets, they buy in quantities that make you think they still had to take the pack mules over the mountains and lay in supplies to last six months. This overbuying quickly translates into waste. According to recent figures, 96 billion pounds of good edible food is wasted in the USA every year. This when people in many parts of the world face hunger, starvation, and lives eked out on a couple of dollars per day.

Why do people in the USA tend to buy far more food than they can possibly eat rather than match purchases to the amount of food needed to maintain their bodies at a healthy, normal weight? There are a number of reasons for this. Some are historical. Some are social. Some can only be explained that for a great many Americans, too much is never enough.

Food shopping habits tend to be passed down from generation to generation. Americans on the frontier, far from stores, had to lay in supplies of necessities they could not provide for themselves. My next-door neighbor, a native South Texan, told me that when he was growing up on a ranch in the Big Bend area, it was 57 miles from his home to the nearest store. Many of us have parents or grandparents who knew the deprivations and hunger of the Great Depression in the 1930s. An overstocked pantry reassures these people. Other Americans keep the freezer and shelves well supplied so to have food on hand in case guests should arrive unexpectedly. Of course "dropping in" unexpectedly is not a French thing to do. Invitations to guests are generally issued well in advance so they can be properly planned and prepared for. Therefore, a French woman can be assured that she only need supply the needs of the family for the meals for which she is shopping.

French homemakers also have a sure sense of how much the family will eat at a meal and buy and prepare only that amount. In France, *restes* (leftovers), unless they are to be incorporated in the next day's meal, are seen as a sign of poor planning and inefficiency on the part of the homemaker. The benefits for weight control: If extra food is not bought and prepared, it is impossible to overeat it.

Shopping for one evening meal in France, can be easy, at least in Paris. Here is Harriet Welty Rochefort, author of *French Toast* describing shopping for the family evening meal in one of her charming Paris Letters on *Paris.org*.

> I just walked down the rue de Poncelet, one of the most wonderful market streets in Paris, and bought our dinner—tarama, tournedos, broccoli, a Brie and a chévre, and a tarte aux pommes. We washed it down with a good Bordeaux and every single member of my family licked his or her lips and concurred that the dinner had been a good one indeed. Food is one of the everlasting ever-present all important good things in a country where savoir-vivre is still alive and well, so I say. . . Vive la France!

In most cities and towns in the USA, Americans, like the French in France, can buy prepared foods and bring them home for a meal. Though in most regions of the USA, instead of taking a brisk walk down some American equivalent of the rue de Poncelet, Americans will be idling the motors of their SUVs in the drive-thru at McDonald's or KFC. They probably won't bring home much tarama, tournedos, or heads of fresh broccoli.

BUYING TOO MUCH

Whether Americans eat carry-out or prepare meals at home, the likelihood is they will bring into the house more food than their bodies need for a healthy, normal weight. When Americans bring this excess food into their homes, there are two things they can do with it: Eat it.

Or throw it out. Many people, unwilling to throw out all that food their hard-earned cash has bought, opt for overeating. Are we surprised that the obesity rates rise?

The basic rule of food shopping for weight control is this: if you don't buy it and bring it home, it won't be in the cupboard or refrigerator when you have an attack of the munchies. I never have much sympathy for someone who says they are trying hard to lose weight and they aren't having success. Yet when I look around their kitchens, I find three pints of ice cream in their freezer and a cupboard overflowing with all sorts of processed snack foods. All the fresh fruits I can find are unripe and with no fruit aroma nor taste. Any low-cal vegetables are withering in plastic bags in the refrigerator humidifier drawer.

If you want to lose weight and stay slim, keep a lean pantry. Make sure most of the food you stock is fresh fruits and vegetables and lean proteins. Keep *junque* food in limited supply. Or don't buy snack foods at all if you have a problem keeping your eating of these items in moderation.

But you say you are not the only person in the household. Others who can eat "anything they please," bring high-calorie snack food into the house and that is what tempts you. Here's a personal solution to that problem.

When my son was growing up, after Halloween and Christmas, he would have candy from his trick or treating and from the various Christmas parties. He has always had the wonderful ability to eat moderately, chew carefully, practice all those good food habits that allow you to eat all sorts of good rich food and stay slim. He would leave his holiday candy on his desk or dresser and eat only a piece or two a day for weeks until it was gone. I discovered to my dismay that, when my son's holiday candy was out in plain sight, I would unconsciously wander into his room and graze on it.

The solution: I asked him to hide the candy from me. Kids love to hide things, so he willingly complied with my request. With the candy out of sight, and since hunting is a conscious activity, Mom,

Candy Kleptomaniac, was no longer mindlessly wandering into his room filching candy snacks.

LOOKING FOR CAUSES

The psychologist Dr. Nathaniel Branden, in my opinion, has prepared the best books and tapes for dealing with the self-esteem issues. (Since self-esteem and weight control are so specifically linked, I recommend Dr. Branden's works to you.) He advises that as adults we have to recognize and make accommodation for "the child we once were." I seemed to have no difficulty with other kinds of candy around the house—say when my mother, an expert candy maker, has given us some of her delicious homemade fudge or that Oklahoma speciality known as Aunt Bill's Brown Candy. When I have a box of Valentine's chocolates, I have no problem eating these in a careful, conscious manner: one piece with a demitasse of after-dinner coffee two or three evenings a week.

My reaction to my son's candy seems a perfect example of what Dr. Branden writes about: that fat child I once was going after the candy even when I, influenced by French women, had successfully made so many other lifestyle changes.

Another example of this involves a cookie jar made for me in the early 1970s by my sister-in-law, a professional potter. The glaze had been toned to match the decor of my kitchen. A beautiful example of the pottery craft, it had to be displayed on the kitchen counter. But I quickly discovered as soon as I put the cookie jar to its intended use, every time I walked through the kitchen, I mindlessly took a cookie from the jar and ate it.

My solution was to leave the cookie jar on the counter, but instead of using it for cookies, I kept my supply of plastic bags in it. I moved the cookies down to a bottom drawer of the kitchen cabinet. I knew the cookies were there, but in that location they did not tempt me. The cookies only tempted me to overeat when they were stored in the same place that they had been stored in my home when I was a child.

When I am a guest in someone's home, I must be on alert I don't begin making unconscious raids on a cabinet top cookie jar. Sometimes I ask my hosts to remove the cookie jar during my visit. I mentioned this problem to my mother on one visit. My next visit I noticed she had a new cookie jar I had never seen before on her kitchen cabinet. She said it was a birthday gift from a friend. For the first couple of days I consciously restrained myself. Then one day I "forgot" and reached into the cookie jar. I found my hand up to the knuckles in whole wheat flour.

SHOPPING DAILY

Probably the biggest difference in food shopping in France and the USA is that French homemakers still shop on a daily or almost-daily basis. As many French women are employed outside the home as women in the USA. Still, most French women continue this traditional system of buying only what the family will consume at the meals eaten before the next shopping. Despite those wonderful restaurants in France, the French still eat about 70 percent of lunches and 90 percent of dinners at home. Since recipe ingredient amounts are listed in weights, and since ingredients are sold by weight, it is possible for French women to buy only enough of the ingredients to prepare the dish they intend to serve.

I have seen, for instance, French women shopping for ingredients for a *gâteau* and carrying a cookbook with them as they shopped. They would ask the shopkeeper for only the exact number of grams of sugar, flour, chocolate, and other ingredients the recipe requires. If the cake called for leavening such as baking powder or baking soda, these are sold in France in small paper packages, allowing you to buy only the amount needed in your recipe. You don't have to buy a whole can of baking powder or a whole box of baking soda as in the USA. This cuts down on the amount of cabinet space needed to store the ingredients. There are no items that you need to use up the rest in making more than you intended. Also, the quality of the dish you prepare will probably be higher since the ingredients are always fresh. They haven't been sitting in your cabinet, growing stale. What American cook has not suffered a baking failure because baking powder or soda has lost its oomph?

THE TYRANNY OF STUFF

In the introduction to this chapter, I explained that my initial reaction to my French friends's fewer material possessions was to feel sorry for them. Yet, I have come to see how having less, but having the right things (a very important qualification), can lead to more efficient and enjoyable living. John Ruskin, the British lifestyle guru of the Victorian era wrote: "Every increased possession loads us with a new weariness." This written by an upper-class English gentleman who employed parlor maids to do the dusting.

Of course, I cannot imagine life without modern appliances, particularly my computer and my microwave, two items, as my life is currently structured, extremely necessary to efficient living and working. The trick: Find what appliances and other material possessions make your life better and which are complicating and frustrating it. I couldn't live without my microwave and I am unwilling to part with a more than 20-year-old counter-top toaster oven, yet I have never owned an electric can opener. I use few canned food products. Certainly not enough to justify the space an electric can opener would take on my kitchen counter. I'd rather use that space for one of my beloved teapots.

When I wrote in the original *Chic&Slim* and posted material on the *Chic&Slim* website about clearing out the excess in your household as a way to cut down housework time (and giving you more time to pamper yourself) and to minimize the frustrations that lead to eating comfort foods, I received emails from women in the USA who thought I was advocating that they give up their much-loved decorator items. They misunderstood.

I am not suggesting you give up treasures. I could not imagine parting with beautiful items full of wonderful associations of people and places that I have collected as I have lived and traveled in various corners of the world. French crystal, German china, Maltese blown glass, English teapots, handmade Indian furniture, African wood carvings, American handmade quilts, Italian pewter, Tunisian tiles, my treasured books, family photos, the boxes of my son's school artwork and writings.

What I am advocating is getting rid of that set of tires out in the garage that only fits a car you sold three years ago, the service for four in pottery taking up space in the kitchen cabinet. You haven't served a meal on those dishes since 1987. Plus the clothes in your closet that are out of style and don't fit, the seven books of unused personal checks to an account you closed last year, advertising brochures and other drawer clutter, worn-out cassettes, cans of dried paint in the garage, out-of-date prescription medicines, as well as the old sweeper you no longer use since you bought a new one.

Things that are taking up space, but contributing nothing to the richness of your life, are what I advocate you clear out.

If your excess items are usable, sell them or give them to someone who needs them. If they can be recycled, do the environment and future generations a good turn and take the stuff to a recycling center. In the case of checks, business cards, dried paint, and outdated prescription medicines, throw them away. Remember some toxic substances cannot go in a regular landfill. Personal information best be shredded.

CLUTTER AUTHORITY ADVICE

Don Aslett, authority on decluttering, writes in *Not For Packrats Only: How to Clean Up, Clear Out, and Dejunk Your Life Forever!* that "Across the board, rich or poor, mansion or bungalow, twelve kids or two, junk and clutter causes more headaches, strained backs, strained budgets, and strained relationships, more frustration, discouragement, guilt, embarrassment, chaos, and confusion than any other housework challenge!" He also reminds us that clutter causes fires and accidents, it attracts vermin and vandals. If your junk is in plain view in your yard, it upsets your neighbors. Don Aslett, by the way, maintains that about 40 percent of "housework" is nothing but picking up and straightening up junk and clutter. You are spending almost half your housework time on stuff you don't need anyway. No wonder French women have time for sitting in sidewalk cafes and for taking their siestas that give them such a beautiful, healthy glow. They are doing less housework because they are organized and don't have the clutter of excess possessions.

Besides, clutter and *junque* are not chic. Your living quarters, your office, and your vehicle are part of your personal style. No matter how chicly dressed you are, if your sink and counter tops are piled with dirty dishes, if your living room is cluttered with piles of unopened junk mail, if your car is littered with empty fast-food containers and advertising flyers, and if your office is in disarray, it will detract from your chic image.

A horrendous description of office clutter was in a *Vanity Fair* article on Esther Dyson, the internationally known high-tech guru. An article photograph caught in graphic detail the guru's Manhattan office. The article's author Leslie Bennetts wrote:

> Immense piles of papers are heaped on every available surface, cascades of stuff overflow every shelf and drawer. Staggering quantities of junk are jumbled three feet deep on every square inch of floor: sweat clothes, stuffed animals, beat-up running shoes, discarded bras, magazines, skin creams and lotions, mountains of newspapers, a plastic container of mayonnaise, teetering stacks of books, tote bags with damp bathing suits trailing out of them, a half-eaten chocolate bar.

Offices are part of personal style, and they make statements about us. Perhaps Esther Dyson is sending a personal style message that, like her office, the cyberworld is a cluttered and messy place, but she can still function effectively and successfully in it. The article quoted a business associate who occupied a nearby office calling Ms. Dyson's clutter "weird and sick."

HOARDING/OVEREATING

If your home is stuffed with clutter, you may be stuffing yourself with too much food just the way you are stuffing your home with too many material items. If I find myself hungry for between-meal snacks, I look around. Often disorder has set in. Usually, putting my home office in order is enough to nick those gnawing mind hunger twinges.

Clutter can divert your concentration. You cannot move as quickly and as safely in a cluttered house. Clutter also makes it more difficult to locate things. Things such as your car keys, the tool you need, or the bill you must pay.

A few years ago I read how many hours per year the average American spends hunting things they have misplaced. I can't remember the exact figure, but it was *days* of time, time that would be much more enjoyable spent in activities such as pampering oneself, or exercising, or spending pleasant hours with friends.

I believe that the French disinclination to clutter living spaces with an oversupply of decorator items and consumer goods is part of French tidy-mindedness. A lot of "stuff" sitting around just can't be neat and organized. More so, excess stuff would cut down on their *joie de vivre*. Part of *savoir-vivre*, knowing how to live, is knowing how much stuff you need to experience the true pleasures of life. And not acquiring more than that amount.

Decide what material items are necessary to the lifestyle that satisfies you. Get rid of those items that keep you from living as well—and as slim as you want. How do you identify the point at which your material possessions aid you in having a satisfying life and a healthier, more attractive body, but beyond which they would complicate and frustrate, and eat up valuable time?

Everyone is unique with unique needs and capacities. As each of us has a different body and state of health and metabolism that allows us to eat more and still stay slimmer than others, so each of us needs different material things and different amounts of material possessions. An American woman Grace Deer wrote in *Sedona Magazine* that she did not believe that more than enough is better than enough. She added that she learned it was not "how big or how much that matters, but how much possessions crowd out the open spaces of the heart."

We know people who are so focused on what they have and on acquiring more that there is no other room left in them. Their possessions, have, as Grace Deer warned, crowded out the open spaces of their hearts.

HOW MUCH IS ENOUGH?

We all know people who have a wealth of material possessions, yet they are caring and giving people whose quantity of possessions in no way hinders their humanity and philanthropy. One thinks of actress Audrey Hepburn, born the daughter of a Dutch baroness, a famous actress, residing in her beautifully furnished seventeenth century Swiss farmhouse surrounded by enchanting gardens, with her Givenchy wardrobe and her jewels. Yet in middle-age, when she could have comfortably remained at home in her lovely Swiss village and tended beautiful gardens, she toured as UNICEF ambassador, acting in behalf of the world's poorest and most destitute children, and traveling to the most primitive parts of the world, viewing the ghastly poverty, deprivation, and disease.

I am quite sure I would not be a better person should I give away the lovely things in my home that give me so much pleasure. Yet I am also quite sure that I would not be happier if I acquired more than I have thus far collected. After several decades of acquiring, some years ago I reached the point where I have enough. In fact, in packing up for a recent move, I became convinced that I have more than enough and I have sold, given away, and thrown away many items that were more a part of my previous lifestyles than the current one.

Just as no one else can prescribe for you what foods you may eat in what quantities and still stay slim, no one can tell you exactly which and how much of the material things of life you need in order to have a happy, satisfying, and slim life. Beyond which those possessions would hinder your pleasure in life.

I received an email from a woman who wrote that after reading *Chic&Slim*: "I decided to move into a smaller, nicer, apt. instead of a larger place for same $. Doing that meant I had to get rid of a lot of stuff I didn't need and didn't want and didn't use, i.e., making room for myself."

I was struck by her phrase "making room for myself." Sometimes "stuff" around us takes up space we really need for ourselves.

Since no one else can tell you what you need and how much of it you need, you must discover this for yourself. French women can give us help with this process. After all, the French certainly could never be considered anti-materialist. For centuries France has produced and sold some of the world's most exclusive luxury goods.

Let's look at how French women decorate and organize their households to give them maximum time for family, friends, beauty treatments, shopping, preparing a healthy cuisine, and that chief French anti-stress activity: sitting in sidewalk cafes.

TIDY HOUSEHOLDS

Of course, the surest way to avoid cluttering your household is not to buy excess stuff in the first place. This is basically the French approach. It is certainly not the American approach. As John Cassidy wrote in "No Satisfaction: The trials of the shopping nation" in *The New Yorker:* "Other nations may have overtaken us in areas like education, manufacturing and public transportation, but they haven't come close to us in the art of zipping around town with a wallet full of plastic."

In the USA, more is the name of the game. But that doesn't necessarily translate into happiness or pleasure on the part of the purchaser. Actually, quite often we don't need more clothes; we need the *right* clothes. We don't need more kitchen equipment; we need the *right* kitchen equipment to prepare quickly and healthily the foods we like to eat on a regular basis. We don't need more men in our lives; we need the *right* man.

French women take time to know themselves. The self-analysis that aids them designing a captivating personal style, also guides them in making the correct purchases for their household. When you spend time shopping for things that you don't need or that don't please or satisfy you, it's a waste of your time that you could be devoting to more pleasurable activities.

As numerous writers and social critics have pointed out, in the USA, abundance often is translated into waste.

The extraordinary thing about waste in the USA is that few Americans realize how truly wasteful they are. Only when you live abroad and return and see the difference in consumption quantities in other countries as compared to the USA do you realize the extremes to which Americans take wasting.

No surprise that houses and landfills are filled to overflowing. Abundance also gets translated into waste of our money, our time, our health, years of our lives just coping with stuff that really doesn't add to the quality of our life.

We need to acquire more intelligently with more planning. We need to choose that which satisfies. And we must cease expecting material things to compensate for our own lack of self-esteem or worthwhile interests. Many American men, hoping to be more successful in the dating arena, might concentrate less on acquiring a sports car and more on washing the outside and vacuuming the inside of the vehicle they do have, on standing up straighter so that their pot belly might not be so obvious, on trimming their nose hairs, and on investing in an over-the-counter product effective against intestinal gas.

SHOPPING TIME

I do not like shopping. Many other activities give more pleasure than looking at merchandise and buying it. I shop when I cannot do without something. I try to buy those things which will give me long service and little frustration. And I try to organize my shopping excursions to make the most efficient use of my time. Here is where a personal style that is based on classics that can be worn for years, rather than the trendy, can cut down substantially on the amount of time needed for clothes shopping.

Like many, I have embraced e-commerce. Buying from online stores allows me to avoid fighting traffic, exposing myself to annoyances and germs, and to eternal waits at the cash register. E-commerce takes away much unpleasantness of conventional shopping and saves time. It also gives me access to products I cannot find locally such as the wonderful teas I buy from online tea merchants.

CLOTHES SHOPPING

In the original *Chic&Slim,* I wrote how clothes shopping is often an unsettling and unhappy process for American women. But buying clothes is a pleasure for French women who achieve such splendid personal styles with small workable wardrobes.

Not long ago, I was in a local store trying on jeans in one of the stalls and feeling pleased that I fit well into pants of a size I could never tugged over my hips when I was a teenager. In the next changing stall were a young mid-twenties mother and her about three-year-old daughter. I heard the woman's voice say with a note of sadness, "This one is too small for Mommy." Sounds came of her removing the garment and putting on another. The child's voice pronounced the verdict. "Too small for mommy." I heard the mother's discouraged sigh. Then fifteen seconds later, she said brightly to the child, "Well, now let's go to Chuck E. Cheese's and eat pizza!"

Whoa! The point of shopping is to buy something that makes you look wonderful today. If you have expanded a bit with pregnancy, or otherwise gained from your teenage weight, then simply try on clothes that are the size you are now and that make you look as good as you can look at your present body shape.

Take at least three sizes of a style you try on into the fitting room. Sometimes I take three pairs of jeans in the *same* size into the fitting room and find that each one is slightly different in hip fit and leg length. French women accept that the fit of pants is very important. They are willing to spend time searching in order to find the pair that looks most flattering to them. Often they go to the expense of alteration to make sure they get the best fit.

Taking several sizes to the fitting room would have increased the chances that the young mother would find something that would make her look attractive—and unlikely to abandon clothes shopping to solace her disappointment in pizza. Besides, what an unfortunate lesson the young mother was giving her daughter. Not only in clothes shopping, but in dealing with disappointment.

I have never dined in a Chuck E. Cheese's establishment, so I am unfamiliar with the menu. But I do hope there is some item on it more friendly than a American-style pizza to a mommy who could not fit into any of the clothes she took into the dressing room. I remember a little French poolside restaurant that served pizza. I always ordered a *Quatre Saisons* (Four Seasons). The crust, baked wonderfully crisp in a brick oven, was topped with a light brush of olive oil and slices of fresh tomatoes, onions, green peppers, and zucchini. The pizza was about six inches in diameter and served without cheese. With a glass of mineral water, that pizza was a very friendly lunch for young mommy figures.

THE VAT

The French have to be more efficient shoppers than Americans. They have the VAT, or Value Added Tax, currently, I believe, at about 18 percent, assessed when one buys consumer items such as appliances, cars, computers, and other luxury items.

We don't have a VAT in the USA, though several individuals, including Cornell University economist Robert Frank, author of *Luxury Fever: Why Money Fails to Satisfy in an Era of Excess,* have proposed such a tax as an alternative to income tax. The French have the VAT *and* the income tax, a tax that every red-blooded Frenchman believes is his civic duty to pay as little as possible.

The VAT, as much as the French insistence on quality, is why if you find an appliance in a French home, it will likely be high quality. An American will say, well, I will just buy this cheapy model and later replace it with something better. A French woman on a budget will likely do without until she can buy the quality version. French women don't want to pay the VAT on an item that won't last a long time.

FRENCH KITCHENS

Earlier, I mentioned how French women generally shop on a daily or almost-daily basis and how they buy only as much as the family can eat. In France, leftovers are frowned upon as evidence of a homemaker's inefficiency and lack of planning.

Naturally, this tendency to keep a minimal amount of food on hand has an effect on the French kitchen. As I wrote in the original *Chic&Slim*, when I first saw French kitchens, I was surprised that they could turn out this legendary French cuisine in such small spaces lacking what I considered the necessary modern equipment. Often, there were no cupboards as we know them in American kitchens. There was sometimes a screened cabinet called a *garde-manger* that would protect the food on hand from insects. Dishes were stored in a china cabinet.

French kitchens of late are becoming more like American kitchens, with larger and more appliances. Previously, French kitchens (city kitchens more than French country kitchens) had been solely for food preparation. Eating was done in another room. Now the French are entertaining in their kitchens.

There are benefits for weight control when kitchens are solely for cooking, and when one course is eaten, the serving dishes are cleared, and excess food is removed to the kitchen. That removes temptation to eat any leftover food, one way I observe Americans consuming extra calories for which they have no true hunger. One can only hope that the French will not let their expanded use of their kitchens keep them in such close proximity to food that they succumb to the temptation to overeat.

I receive emails in which women ask if the French habit of daily shopping will work well in the United States. For a great many of us, the answer is no. Daily food shopping is one French technique for staying chic and slim that does not translate well to American life. To test it, when I was writing the original *Chic&Slim*, I spent one week, seven days, when I shopped once daily for only what I would eat in the next 24-hour period. That turned out to be a real time eater for someone who works in a home office, as I do. And I lived only a short one-half-mile drive from an H-E-B Food Store, which I consider the most innovative and customer-oriented supermarket chain in the world.

Why does the daily shopping work so well for the French? For one thing, they are going out anyway twice, if not three times a day, to buy that fresh baked French bread. They tend to live in apartments in city centers so that all the shops are handily nearby. They usually patronize neighborhood shops and produce stalls. They are more accustomed to walking to shopping. Too, the French believe that freshly cooked, well-prepared food is so essential to the pleasure of life that they are willing to put out the effort needed to purchase food as fresh as possible.

I received an email from a American woman who was making her system of shopping only three times per week work for her. She wrote:

Three years ago I began to shop for groceries three times a week. I shop on Monday, Wednesday, and Friday. This is the most wonderful way to shop, no wonder the French shop frequently! I only buy enough food to get my family to the next shopping day. For instance, on Monday I only buy what we will need until Wednesday, etc. I no longer have to throw out leftovers or extra foods in the freezer that weren't used right away. My refrigerator and freezer are neat and clean!!! I have found that I don't spend as much money in the long run either (even though I no longer buy the large bonus packs of food). The best part is that I'm in the store only about 10 minutes and can usually go through the 12 items or less checkout AND I don't have to spend a half hour unloading my car and restocking my cabinets. I highly recommend this technique!!! It takes a little getting used to but is worth every bit of the effort.

Three times a week seems far more practical than every day. But, as far as living chic and slim goes, what is important is not the number of times a week you shop, as what best suits your lifestyle. The best schedule for you will depend on your work schedule, your distance from food shopping, the type of food shopping available to you, the size of your family, what style meals you prepare, the season. (In bad weather, when driving to the store might be difficult or dangerous, you would want to keep more food on hand.)

What is most important is that you not overbuy food so that you find yourself either overeating or wasting. Having lived in countries where children regularly cry themselves to sleep at night because they are hungry, I have a real problem with people who waste edible food. Buy only what you can eat, and donate the money you did not spend on food you would throw away to the Salvation Army, your local food bank, or UNICEF.

The system of buying only enough for meals until you next shop will work better if you have a routine. French women are strong on routine. This simplifies their lives and cuts down on stress. Unfortunately, in the USA, being organized is often looked on with suspicion. If you aren't rushed and exhausted, if your life is not in constant crisis, well, you must not be really trying. If you are organized, you risk being labeled obsessive. Or neurotic or eccentric. In the USA, being organized and in control of your life is often seen as a disease, not a virtue. Alas.

The advantages to an ordered life, however, seem to me to far outweigh the minor inconvenience of a few tacky comments by people who are jealous.

FAD FOODS
Something else helps the French keep a neat, uncluttered kitchen. The French are eating three and a half decades later much the same diet that they were eating when I first began observing them. True, some French restaurants went through a period of Nouvelle Cuisine, but at-home fare remained the traditional *Cuisine Bonne Maman* or *Cuisine Bonne Femme*. Good old traditional French home cooking.

But what a difference from the USA, where people are continually adopting and discarding food fads. I noticed this especially when I was living abroad and only returning for visits every two years or so. One trip back, everyone seemed to be making Reuben Meatloaf, a Reuben sandwich converted to a baked casserole. The next trip, Reuben Meatloaf was only a memory preserved in bloating cans of sauerkraut on pantry shelves. The new fad recipe would be concocted from canned fruit cocktail and whipped topping. This highly sugared dish I was horrified to find served as the salad. Salad! What happened? I would ask. Did a freeze kill the lettuce?

In the USA, each food fad has its day, then is forgotten. Cabinets clutter with the spring-form pans, tandoori dishes, and unused jars of wasabi sauce. The French keep eating the same dishes they ate decades ago, preparing them in their one or two well-used pots hanging from hooks over the kitchen stove. The authors of *French Style* write: "Americans, though aware of the French concern of gourmet food, tend to be surprised by the simplicity of most French kitchens and charmed by the age and authenticity of century-old furniture and fixtures."

Cooking the same dishes for decades has advantages. When you do the same thing in the same way for a long time, you usually become efficient at the task. You have the equipment you need. So for Christmas your gift can be a lacy nightgown instead of Calphalon cookwear. When you cook the same things that you have cooked many years, then, shopping and meal preparation becomes more automatic, easier, quicker, and less stressful. You have more time and more serenity in your life. Life is more pleasurable. And you will likely be slimmer. Not just because of less stress in your life, but for the practical reason that if you are always trying out new recipes you tend to take in extra calories tasting your efforts. A dish you have cooked for years does not require taste tests.

DECORATING STYLE

In *French Style*, the wonderful book on French interior decoration by Suzanne Slesin, Stafford Cliff, and Jacques Dirand, the Paris-based designer Andrée Putman explains French reverence for the old, and how it is rare in France to begin decorating a house with new items. "There is always an aunt, godmother, or grandfather to give us a dresser or a table service. And if not, there are flea markets from which we can invent a past."

Mme Putman explains the French throw nothing away and how shocked they are when in the USA they find abandoned furniture out for the trash pickup, something one would *never* see in France.

Like the French, my family never throws away a piece of furniture. My son has dubbed the attic of my mother's spacious old house as the Family Furniture Archives. I have acquired some nice pieces from those archives, and from discards from friends who tend to redecorate frequently.

Andrée Putnam also describes what she finds as the best in French decoration style. She describes a house that is alive and free and that is an extension of the personal style of the inhabitants of that house. These homes have charm, spontaneity, and eclecticism. She says that this "tendency toward the casual is nothing other than elegance."

FRENCH BATHROOMS

One room in the house in which the French were long known for revering (and not replacing) the old was the bathroom. But French plumbing, like French telephones, no longer deserve the antiquated, poorly functioning reputation they held for so long. Some of the descriptions of plumbing encountered in the last few years in France sound positively futuristic.

One appliance essential to the French bathroom not commonly found in American bathrooms is the bidet. I wrote about this fixture for "localized cleansing" in the original *Chic&Slim*. From some of the responses, I learned that the bidet was becoming more popular in the United States. In fact, it was suggested that I might like to housesit for one family during their absence strictly because they had a bidet. The friend who suggested the housesitting thought I might be missing the appliance.

I also learned that if you have acquired the habit of using a bidet when living in France, it is possible to purchase various gadgets that fit over a conventional American commode so that it can be used for the bidet function. This may give the impression that bidets have become more popular with Americans than they actually are. My American friends who found bidets in the French-built homes they occupied quite often found alternative uses for them. One filled the bidet with pots of house plants. My friend said that the fountain in the center that provides the cleaning spray when seated upon it made a wonderful way to shower the plants with water. Another friend found her bidet useful for filling with water and washing out her hand laundry. Still another family used it as a home for pet goldfish. Another as a terrarium for a small turtle.

My favorite bidet was one, like the tub, basin, and commode in my bathroom, made of a pale rose petal pink porcelain. Quite lovely and feminine, I thought. *Très* French.

DECORATING FRENCH STYLE

The French approach to decorating is: begin with a few pieces and slowly add items you love that have meaning for you. Some years ago, I read that items decorating a French home were, for all practical purposes, icons. For all of us who decorate with meaningful items, those items are icons of sorts. Surely another reason for getting rid of the clutter: so we can enjoy to the fullest those things around us that we love and which have meaning. Enjoy our icons without the distraction of useless junk.

But how to keep down clutter? I had a great aunt who had a system for gifts. She kept a minimalist household and the leanest closet I have ever seen—and she was consistently well dressed. When you gave her a gift, she wrote you a thank you note. The next time you visited, she gave you back all the gifts you had sent her since you last visited. Her system of returning gifts added a new dimension to choosing a gift you liked yourself. She herself always gave gifts in the form of a check. To my way of thinking, checks are the most considerate gifts. They allow recipients to buy precisely what they need and want. I can remember times of great financial hardship in my life when I was given expensive, impractical gifts for which I had absolutely no need. Heartbreaking.

LEAN CLOSET FOR A LEAN BODY

French women are known as the best-dressed women in the world. Surprisingly, they earn this title with small, well-planned wardrobes. Even more surprising is the fact that they are experts at achieving their chic without spending a fortune. Many French women simply do not have much income to devote to clothes. Their chic requires hunting the best possible prices and making wise long-term fashion investments.

French women use these small, well-planned wardrobes to help them stay slim. For one thing, if you have only a small number of good quality clothes that fit you like a glove, you don't dare gain a half-kilo or you will have nothing to wear.

If you have an overstuffed closet, it may be contributing to your difficulties to stay slim. Especially if there are clothes in the closet that you plan to diet to fit.

On the topic of keeping clothing that is too small, I received the following email written in response to another email posted on the website in which a woman bemoaned no success in her weight-loss efforts. In the responding email, Virginia wrote:

> I am 5'6" tall and look really awful even at 140. 145-150 is my ideal weight, and I can carry it because I work out (very moderately, not to bulk up) and because of my basic body build. And yet, "society" would have me and others like me believe that I am bordering on obese and should be locked up with no food until I reach an "acceptable" weight of 125. Ridiculous.

Remember that muscle weighs five times more than fat. So a body with little excess fat will weigh more than one the same size that is not so well-toned. That is why body measurements are more important than numbers on the scale.

Virginia went on to write that once she realized that she could be healthy and attractive at the weight that was right for her, coping with stress-provoked overeating became easier. She continued:

> By the way, I got rid of anything in my closets that didn't fit. I was haunted by some very small clothes that—following a starvation regimen and before I got smart about my body and its needs—I still kept, hoping I'd get back into them. Loved your tip on cleaning out our closets!

BOUDOIRS FOR SLIM

Many Americans are confused in their understanding of a boudoir and its purpose. The confusion is understandable because boudoirs have played different roles in different historical times. Today, they offer a woman a sanctuary and refuge from pressures of modern life. They are a place to recover from stress and pamper oneself.

Boudoirs are a French conception. The word itself comes from the French verb *bouder,* which means "to sulk or to pout." In the early 17th century, a young French noblewoman, the Marquise de Rambouillet, didn't think men should have all the fun of evenings of intellectual discussions that excluded women. She remodeled her mansion near the Louvre so that it contained several large reception rooms, or *salons.* To these salons she invited the liveliest minds. In her *chambre bleue,* she received visitors from her bed. Gary Kamiya wrote in "A Brief History of Salons" on *Salon.com,* "It may seem odd that discussion groups led by middle-age French society women from their bedrooms should have had a decisive influence on Western civilization. It was the civilizing influence of women upon ordinarily dogmatic and combative men that allowed the French salon to change the course of intellectual history."

That was one sort of boudoir. Another is that portrayed in the French theater productions the so-called "bedroom farces." But the modern sort of boudoir that helps French women stay serene and slim is one where she can be alone and have an opportunity to restore herself from life's innumerable stresses.

In the original *Chic&Slim,* I quoted writer Judith Thurman's description of her French friend's boudoir in her Parisian apartment. The small room with its marble fireplace and French doors opening onto a tiny balcony trailing ivy and geraniums (how Parisian!) sounded like the perfect place to seclude oneself and read, or simply watch rain fall.

For those women who live alone, the need today is not so much to have a boudoir in their living quarters as to set aside a "boudoir time." For this half hour or so, you need to disconnect yourself from all the modern connections that today give us no moments of stillness.

Thomas Friedman, author of *The Lexus and the Olive Tree: Understanding Globalization* calls overconnectedness the social disease of the 21st century. With our cellphones, our faxes, our technology, we are now connected to the whole world no matter where are. "Out is over. Now, you're always in. And when you're always in, you're always on. And when you're always on, you're just like a computer server. You can never stop and relax." I would add that when you can never be "off," eventually the circuits are going to overheat and you are going to burn out.

Take a daily "boudoir time." Take at least a half hour a day when you turn off your phone, your cellphone, your pager, your fax machine, whatever beeps to tell you that you have new email. Ignore your doorbell. Spend some time with yourself and you will be more ready to spend time with those you care about. You will surely find it easier to lose weight and stay slim.

AFTERNOON TEA

For me, the best boudoir activity is afternoon tea. The writer Henry James said, "There are few hours in life more agreeable than the hour dedicated to the ceremony known as afternoon tea." I agree. Those of you who regularly visit *annebarone.com*, the companion to my *Chic&Slim* books, know my devotion to this civilized custom. I depend on afternoon tea for daily restoration and maintenance of my sanity.

We think of afternoon tea as an English custom, but the French, I love to point out, were having afternoon tea a century before Anna, Duchess of Bedford, began the practice in England. Madame de Sévigné wrote of *le thé de cinq heures* (five o'clock tea) long before Anna started passing around tea and scones to stave off hunger till the late dinner hour. This 17th century French tea lover, by the way, is the same Madame de Sévigné who commented, "The more I see of men, the more I admire dogs."

The British actress Elizabeth Hurley explained afternoon tea's beneficial effects for weight control. The British actress was quoted in the January 2000 issue of *Elle*:

But for Hurley, the most important meal of the day comes between four and five. "I have to have a cup of tea, a sandwich, a scone. One of the keys to thinness—and I'd like to share this with the readers of *Elle*—is to have something at tea time. Otherwise you're so hungry and bad-tempered by dinner you either eat the bread basket or have too many drinks."

Afternoon tea is a lovely way to pamper and restore yourself. This works either in teashop or home. Remember to eat chicly.

GARDEN/YARD

Several years ago, I had an American neighbor who hated mowing his lawn and doing other yard-related chores more than anyone I have ever known. Given his feelings on the matter, I was always puzzled why he did not hire someone to mow his lawn; he could well have afforded it. One day, spotting me on my terrace having tea, he called over to me: "Do you know what I really hate about yard work? It doesn't make any money."

My neighbor was right. Lawns do not make money; lawns cost money—and effort. Unlike vegetable gardens, they do not produce anything edible. (Unless you harvest your dandelions for salad.) The French are smarter than people in the USA when it comes to grass and lawns. They never developed the kind of suburban developments that sprawled across the American landscape, trying to give every family, no matter how humble, their own mini-estate.

The French rarely commute long distances. They live close to their work. Or work close to their home. The French have sent the lower-income segment of the population out to the high-rise housing projects in the suburbs. The more affluent have remained in apartments in the city centers, close to the theaters, restaurants, museums, and shops. And they have allowed their law enforcement to keep walking to all these cultural amenities safe. Those tolerate-no-nonsense gendarmes in twos and on foot, keep the streets secure. When the French want grass, trees, and flowers, they go to a park that some civil servant keeps beautiful. Or they go to their weekend homes in the countryside.

French women are realistic. They know French men prefer many things more than yard work. When the French have a yard, it's usually graveled, not grass. Because they love fresh produce, the French will devote an area to a *potager*, a kitchen garden of vegetables, herbs and flowers.

HOME SWEET HOME IN FRANCE

The French have a different criteria for choosing where they live than Americans Louis-Bernard Robitaille explains in his book *And God Created The French*. The Parisian elite's preference for discreet comfort means that the truly chic parts of Paris are not necessarily the most opulent or the most expensive, or even the most striking. He writes:

> When it can afford it (Parisian *Bonne Societé*), sets itself up in a lovely apartment dating, from, say, the eighteenth or nineteenth century, and in the noble part of the seventh arrondissement, the venerable Faubourg Saint-Germain. In utter simplicity. A hundred and fifty square metres, sometimes much less. You find Parisian celebrities and intelligentsia installed in relatively restricted quarters, where at times one must push aside piles of books and pull out the table in order to serve dinner for eight.

CLEANOUT FOR SLIM

Psychologist Belleruth Naparstek's excellent *Weight Loss* guided imagery tape sums up the ways you make progress toward losing weight and staying slim: ". . . you are cleaning out the overstuffed closets of your heart, your mind, your house, your body, your life. . ."

The point is not to make your life devoid of material things, but to put material things in balance with the intellectual and spiritual aspects of your life.

President Theodore Roosevelt in his Thanksgiving Proclamation of 1908 declared:

> For the very reason that in material well-being we have thus abounded, we owe it to the Almighty to show equal progress in moral and spiritual things . . . The things of the body are good;

the things of the intellect better; the best of all are the things of the soul; for, in the nation as in the individual, in the long run it is character that counts.

Character counts in weight control, too. You must be honest with yourself about what you have been doing that keeps you fat before you can begin the process of becoming slim. When you have the material, intellectual, and spiritual parts of your life in balance, you have a better chance of living chic, slim, and happy.

Some material possessions are necessary for successful living. Beyond food, shelter, transportation, health care, safety, we need things to feed our intellect. Something must fill your spiritual needs so you do not fill with food an emptiness inside you.

French women maintain lean kitchen cupboards and clothes closets. Their homes are uncluttered and decorated with revered possessions. They are organized for efficient housekeeping that gives them time to pamper themselves, prepare wonderful meals, and have time for their families. All this pays dividends in chic, svelte bodies.

What is French women's incentive for perfecting their art of being women and their efficient household management? Men. Relationships are important to French women and they help to keep them chic and slim. *Les hommes,* men, make it all worth the effort. In the next chapter we look at how relationships work to keep French women slim.

CHIC & SLIM SUCCESS STORY

Dear Anne,

It's been about a year since I first obtained your book, and I wanted to tell you of my success in improving my self image and loosing weight. I took off 20 lbs. last year and kept it off through the year. I also changed how I look at myself, and started dressing like the sexy, beautiful woman my husband thinks I look like.

I love the ideas you present about eating and self confidence & image. I love the thought that pampering ourselves with a taste of something yummy & decadent is not wrong, and that we will feel better for not feeling so deprived. I love the thoughts you present about the basic differences in men & women, and how the American society is sabotaging us. It's so nice to read about ideas that support what I've always felt were correct but not expressed in this culture.

— *Francesca in Colorado*

CHIC & SLIM

Staying slim is not about counting calories or fat grams. Staying slim is not about exercise exhaustion. Staying slim is really about personal style.

Be chic, Stay slim

Anne Barone
Chic & Slim ✤ *annebarone.com*

6

L'AMOUR & LA VIE

LOVE. LIFE. AND WEIGHT. WHY ARE RELATIONSHIPS in France better than elsewhere? Why do those good relationships have positive benefits for weight control? How do their relationships keep French women slim?

Louis-Bernard Robitaille wrote in his chapter on French women in his book *And God Created The French*:

> I don't think France is a country that is particularly unfair to women. On the contrary, overall their status in society and their relations with the opposite sex place them less at a disadvantage than most anywhere else. Françoise Giroud, former (French) Secretary of State for the Rights of Women, wrote not long ago that these relations were 'among the most delightful in the world,' which may seem overly enthusiastic, but not far from the truth.

In the original *Chic&Slim*, I began the chapter on French relationships with a statement by Françoise Giroud, that noted writer and former editor of French *Elle*. Mme Giroud had, previously, told Sanche de Gramont, author of *The French,* that France is the only country in the world where men and women really understand each other.

Having observed couples from many countries and cultures, including many French couples, I agree with Mme Giroud. In France men and women do seem to understand each other well. I sensed a spirit of collaboration to make life as pleasurable as possible. Even when times or situations were difficult.

Françoise Giroud did not claim French relationships are idyllic. She admits their problems. Even so, they are better than relationships in the USA. "Combative" and "contentious" are two words often used to describe American relationships. A character in Diane Johnson's novel *Le Divorce* describes them: strained toleration and active dislike.

I believe a chief factor in success of French relationships is French women's practicality. French women accept French men as they *are*. Women in the USA have this notion of how men *should be* and try to devise strategies for changing men to their idealized vision.

Most visions of men as they *should be* ignore realities of history, culture, psychology, and male biology.

For their efforts to redesign men, American women often become exasperated and frustrated. Often, American women seek solace for their, frustration in comfort foods. Too often, their frustration results in conflict and contention. Observers, particularly men who have enjoyed relationships with French women, say that those relationships are less competitive and combative than those with American women.

Why is this? Several factors play a role here.

THE SPORTS MENTALITY PROBLEM

In the USA, the sports mentality pervades every aspect of the culture. The French, however, are more likely to see a relationship as a synergistic partnership in which a woman will give care and acknowledgement, and in return, will receive those small, considerate gestures that so delight the female heart. Far too often, American relationships become a contest in which one partner has to win and the other has to lose. Scores are kept.

The French love sports, too. The Tour de France, the Grand Prix, the Vendée Globe, and the French Open are all wonderful contests for which the entire country shows great interest and enthusiasm. Yet, when it comes to relationships between men and women, romance is prized more highly than competition. The advantage of romance over competition is that both parties in the relationship come out winners. If you did apply a sports mentality to French relationships, it would be that a man and a woman in a relationship are on the same team.

In that previously mentioned Paris-set novel *Le Divorce*, the author Diane Johnson puts forth an interesting analysis of the connection between the relationships between men and women in the USA and weight control. She writes that, in contrast to the cooperation that exists between the sexes in France, in the USA, a state of war exits where everyone gets fat from despair and hostility in order to erotically deprive their loved one.

The theory of American gain weight as a hostile action toward spouses and significant others is interesting. I also suspect that frequently the deep-seated motivation behind some American women's weight gain is that they fear if they are slim and attractive, they will be tempted to have an affair. They think as long as they are unattractive, no one is going to make them "an offer they can't refuse." Both motivations strike me as self-defeating.

A woman might gain weight in order to make herself unattractive to her partner or to keep herself from temptation, but in doing so, she is endangering her health and inflicting the damage to her self-esteem that invariably comes when a woman looks in the mirror and sees a fat, lumpy body. In the first motivation, if her partner becomes disgusted and leaves, if she's overweight, that excess weight will hinder her chances of establishing a relationship with another man with whom she would be happier. In the second, she might keep herself from temptation, but the deterioration in her appearance may put stresses on the relationship she is trying to preserve.

CIVILITY

I am quite certain that another reason French relationships are less combative is the general level of civility (and formality) that still exists in French society. Civility and formality in American culture probably never came anywhere near the *comme il faut* (as it should be) that guides so much French behavior. France is also still a class-conscious society in which people tend to socialize in their own restricted groups. You might have seen the same woman who had an appointment at the same Parisian podiatrist at the same time as you for years. You would have probably exchanged polite greetings and even participated in light conversation. But it would not be unusual that you had not introduced yourselves.

Introductions to new friends come from established friends from within your own social set. Many Americans would interpret this reluctance to socialize outside established groups as preventing making friends with interesting people you might enjoy. The French would more likely interpret it as saving you the annoyance of social contact with someone who does not share your interests and value system. An advantage to socializing within your restricted group is that, in the long run, it keeps social dealings freer from stress. For weight control, of course, less stress is beneficial.

NO SECOND HELPINGS

Another way in which French etiquette aids weight control is in the matter of second helpings. The French, of course, still eat their meals in courses. A meal would begin with an hors d'oeuvre, then comes the main course, salad, cheese, fruit. It is simply bad manners to take a second helping of the hors d'oeuvre, salad, cheese, or fruit courses. A dessert is invariably served as one small portion. *C'est tout!*

Civility and good manners do make life more pleasurable. And remember, pleasure is a chief goal in French life. So, with this emphasis on pleasure, it is no surprise the French are known for good manners. *Savoir-vivre*, knowing how to live, requires knowing correct behavior in all situations. The French have very specific etiquette guidelines to follow. One book, *Guide du Protocole et des Usages.* (Protocol is obvious, but usages might translate into English as "properly done things.") This etiquette bible by Jacques Gandouin is almost 600 pages of specific instructions for behavior.

Another book on French etiquette, one not quite so lengthy, is Christine Géricot's *Le Savoir-Vivre Aujourd'hui* (Knowing How To Live Today). Mme Géricot is very specific on proper behavior in situations involving men and women. For one thing, she is adamant that the man *always* pays for the meal in a restaurant.

The toleration French women demonstrate for much male behavior surprises and infuriates many American women. Male casualness of dress, for one thing. French women manage to look as if they stepped off the cover of a fashion magazine. But the men! For years I thought there must be a French law that prohibited French men from combing their hair. As for washing it, surely there was a universal water shortage that restricted the frequency of that activity. The stereotyped image of the French male, not too clean, in wrinkled clothing, with a cigarette dangling from lips curled into a scowl, is not far from reality.

As for men helping with household chores, that is not much done in France. As I have said elsewhere, I long ago decided that the reason French bathrooms did not have many towel racks was that French women did not expect their husbands to pick up wet towels anyway. Living in apartments frees French men from many of the chores (cleaning out the garage and yard work) that American women nag husbands to perform.

HISTORICAL FACTORS

Historical reasons help explain why French women are so willing to please men by their appearance and attitude, why they are willing to try and make the lives of their husbands and lovers especially pleasurable. By the end of World War I, nearly two million French men were dead out of a population of 10 million men of military age. (That was about 20 percent of the male population of military age and about 10 percent of the total French male population.) Heaviest casualties were suffered by the youngest soldiers: about 30 percent of those drafted from 1912 to 1915. Many of those young men were not yet married. Still, at the end of the war in 1918, there were 630,000 war widows in France. The war deprived a large number of younger French women of the chance of ever marrying. The imbalance between the sexes between 20 and 40 was particularly high. World War II, the Algerian conflict, and the French war in Indochina also killed and mutilated large numbers of French men. A low birthrate contributed to the imbalance in male and female population. Most of the 20th century, French men were in short supply.

So I understand the tolerance French women demonstrate toward French men's foibles. American men died in wars and conflicts of the 20th century, but never in numbers that put men in such noticeably short supply. Perhaps if men were scarcer in the USA, there would be less argument, conflict, and contention in American relationships. Then again, probably not.

THE ARGUMENT CULTURE

Deborah Tannen, an expert on miscommunication and author of *The Argument Culture: Moving From Debate to Dialogue,* claims that misunderstanding is endemic in American culture because many Americans believe the best way to a common goal is by arguing our differences as loudly as possible. We see political talk shows where all the participants shout at once and it is impossible to understand what any are saying. To me, these shows are the mud wrestling of politics. According to Deborah Tannen, what gets lost in the shouting is thoughtful debate and real understanding.

Larissa MacFarquhar in reviewing *The Argument Culture* for *The New York Times Book Review*, wrote that Deborah Tannen's suggestion for replacing shouted arguments with workable ways of negotiating our differences missed an important point. "What Tannen is missing is that conflict is fun. We love fighting for its own sake, even when one side is obviously wrong."

Are arguments between men and women really fun? Really?

Are they fun when medical research has shown that abrasive marital conflicts lower wives's immune function, leading to illness, while their husbands don't suffer poorer health or even feel less happily married? Are they fun when the resulting illness makes it more difficult for women to care for their husband and children and to find the energy to prepare and eat healthy food and to get the exercise needed to stay slim and attractive? Is it fun when diminished self-esteem from the eroded attractiveness causes even more stress and unhappiness?

Are arguments fun when a husband or partner hurls derogatory comments about a woman's body, telling her that she is unattractive and repulsive? Is it fun when men justify their inattentions, infidelities, even their physical abuse on the grounds of a woman's deficiencies in her appearance or her unsatisfying sexual performance?

Can we categorize as "fun" the psychological damage done to children who must witness their parents' shouting matches? Is it fun when these arguments are a prelude to physical violence against women when, according to a recent study done by Dr. Jeanne McCauley, a physician at Johns Hopkins Bayview Medical Center, domestic violence is a leading cause of death and injury to women in the United States?

BOUNDARIES & DISCRIMINATION

I have no idea as to the solution to domestic violence in the USA or elsewhere. Though I am certain that continuing to model relationships on sports contests and war is not useful.

I have had absolutely no experience with physical abuse from a male. Perhaps this is in part due to the model for relationship conduct I learned from French women. For one thing, these boundaries that French women set around themselves (and for which they are often accused of being snobbish or haughty) help a woman avoid relationships that might put her at risk.

Additionally, women who make the effort for an attractive appearance are generally able to be more selective about the men with whom they become involved. (Not that attractive women always make the wisest choices.) Desperation does not drive attractive women to unwise relationships as often as it does the less attractive.

Women who have choices in the men with whom they become involved are also less likely to make excuses for men whose behavior suggests they might be abusive. Use common sense. Enter cautiously into relationships. Acquire enough education and job skills so that if, despite your precautions, you end up in a abusive relationship, you never have to stay in that relationship out of economic desperation. Also use reasonable precaution that you do not inadvertently provoke some man not particularly prone to violence to strike you.

The closest I ever came to having a man hit me happened when I lived in Corpus Christi, Texas. I was taking a walk. Just as I passed a battered pickup truck parked in front of an apartment building, a beer can hit the pavement. Now I feel *very* strongly about littering. So I detoured from my path, picked up the beer can, marched over to the door on the driver's side of the pickup, and said, "Excuse me!" The man was clearly not expecting to have his jettisoned beer container returned to him by an Anne Barone-type of person, so I gained some advantage from my surprise appearance. I poked the beer can in his direction and said, "I am sure that you want to dispose of this *properly.*" He grabbed the can, and for about ten seconds, it looked as if he was going to dispose of that beer can right up my nose. Instead, he threw the beer can into the bed of his truck.

EXPERTS AT HANDLING MEN

John Fairchild, the publisher of *Women's Wear Daily* and *W* who lived many years in France and observed French and European women there, said, "European women, especially Frenchwomen, win hands down for their intelligence in their relationships with men. Deep down they control their men, letting them run free up to a point, then exerting their charm and beauty to see they stay in line."

Please note that John Fairchild said French women use "charm and beauty" to keep their men in line. He did not say nagging, nor arguments. Nor lawsuits.

French women know that men are very visually oriented. Men like to look at attractive women. French women put enormous effort into making themselves attractive, alluring, and exuding feminine appeal to men. French women spend years developing their charm, that indefinable quality that draws someone to you and makes them want to please you and do what you want.

When charm and beauty aren't enough, French women have an effective little technique for getting men to behave as they want them to behave. That's the famous French pout.

THE ART OF THE POUT

You find an excellent lesson in the art of the French pout in the Meg Ryan and Kevin Kline film *French Kiss*. In fact, the whole movie is a textbook in differences in French and American women and their different approaches to handling men.

French pouting has several advantages over American contentious arguments. First, no woman looks her most attractive in a screaming rage. Anger contorts and distorts the face. Mouth gapes open, nostrils flare, all sorts of lines mar the face. Voice is loud and often takes on raucous, unpleasant tones.

The French pout is more alluring—and effective. In a proper pout, the face is arranged quite prettily. One simply and firmly directs one's attention elsewhere from the man you are with. Perhaps to another man. Thus, the pouter may be able to arouse her man's territorial instincts. He will be more willing to come to her terms if he thinks another male is about to claim her. Pouting lips are in perfect position to be kissed when the proper male apologies have been duly offered and—after a strategic length of time—accepted and a reconciliation achieved.

Because a pout is silent, there are no hurled accusations, derogatory remarks, nor insults to regret later and to leave their scars on a relationship. In the French pout, a French woman has simply made herself unavailable to the man for a time, yet remaining in sight, looking wonderfully attractive, and subtly suggesting that her charms might soon be diverted to another.

Two facts about men French women never forget: men are charmed by an attractive appearance and men are territorial. French women put these facts to good use. Perfect your pout.

FEMININITY

Another tool for relationship success French women employ is their femininity. French women have a reputation for being *plus femme*, literally "more woman" than any others in the world. *Les Parisiennes* are so far out in front of the pack that they are in a class by themselves. French women manage to be feminine no matter whether they are racing sailboats, sunning on a Riviera beach, a physician making hospital rounds, hiking in the Alps, or working in a cheese shop.

An interesting comment on French femininity appeared in P.T. Deuterman's marine adventure novel *Scorpion in the Sea: The Goldsborough Incident*. The protagonist says:

> He could not figure out what it was that made her so attractive—she was not beautiful in the conventional sense of the word, but she had a physical, utterly feminine presence unlike any American woman he had met. He was reminded of the French women he had encountered in his travels, who always seem to project an almost blatant femininity before he noticed anything else about them.

When you hear someone say that chic French women are so feminine, what are some of the elements that bring out this much-admired quality? Following is a cursory and incomplete, but I hope useful, list.

First of all, there is French women's priority for skin care. They take great pains to keep their skin smooth and soft.

Second, when they dress, even if they are wearing leggings topped with a man's shirt or sweater (usually commandeered from a man's closet), they wear it in a way that calls attention to some womanly feature—often some erotic feature. Yet they keep that call of attention well within the bounds of good taste.

No matter how tailored or severe their outfit, French women always add one feminine accessory. A decorative brooch on the lapel of a tailored suit, or pretty ribbon tying back the hair when they wear jeans with boots.

One example I used earlier in the book that demonstrates a feminine accessory was the French woman astronaut wearing a pretty strand of pearls with her flight jacket.

Throughout Harriet Welty Rochefort's book *French Toast: An American in Paris Celebrates the Maddening Mysteries of the French*, she gives examples of French women's feminine traits. For instance, speaking in a soft, modulated voice that is a pleasure to the ear, as well as the dainty "tinkle of a laugh" that is acceptable laughter for French women. Loud, sidesplitting guffaws on the part of women are much frowned on in France.

French women don't refill their own wine glass, they always leave that to men. In the USA, alas, many women would become teetotalers by default if they sat around waiting for a man to refill their wine glass.

When a guest in someone's home, a woman (or man) never asks the location of the bathroom. One does not call attention to bodily needs. Though most French seem willing to discuss sexual matters frankly, should the need for a bathroom in someone else's home arise, one discreetly excuses oneself and hunts the proper room. Children sometimes take pity on you and point out the W.C. (Pronounced "dooble-vay-say," the French rendition for the British "water closet.") Thankfully, most French living quarters are small. Even a solo search usually will not take long.

THE UBIQUITOUS HIGH HEEL

Probably the most decidedly feminine apparel with which chic French women declare their femininity are those high-heeled shoes that they determinedly wear, even for quick trips to the bakery, for walking the dog, as footwear at the swimming pool and other places where American women would likely opt for the greater comfort of flat or low heels.

Katell Le Bourhis, an elegant Parisienne, is a former curator of the Costume Institute at the Metropolitan Museum of Art in New York and fashion advisor for Louis Vuitton, the French luxury-good company. The opening paragraph in an *Elle Decor* profile of Katell Le

Bourhis is a wonderful explanation of the chic French woman's feeling about high heeled footwear.

"'I love pointed, pointed, pointed, narrow, narrow, narrow,' says Katell Le Bourhis, throwing one shapely foot high in the air to reveal a midnight-blue Dior satin shoe with the skinniest of ankle straps and the most precipitous of heels. It's the sort of shoe podiatrists would like to see banned. 'I don't care if they make my feet hurt all over—I love the way they make you walk differently,' she says, briefly demonstrating her undulating totter."

An alluring walk is very important to a chic French woman. You can't walk sexy in sneakers. You need proper footwear that also makes your feet look tiny and elegant. Unfortunately, the more overweight you are, the more difficult it is to wear high heels. Excess weight in a number of women I know has contributed to knee and joint problems that restricted them to the flattest, clunkiest, most unsexy shoes. Those high-heeled shoes favored by chic French women are an inducement for them to eat moderately and stay slim so they can continue wearing shoes that give them the sexy feet and walk that men so admire.

French women wear high heels in situations you think they would not. I was astounded French women even wore high heels with swim suits at the pool. Then I remembered that you never saw Miss America come down the runway in shower thongs.

A couple of years ago, I was watching France's Bastille Day parade on television. As is customary in France, the police chiefs march in this parade as a body. There are few female police chiefs in France, but one was prominently in view front row right flank. All the male police chiefs were wearing their regular uniforms and sturdy boots. The female chief wore her uniform jacket with a knee-length skirt (that revealed her attractive legs), and, of course, high-heeled dress pumps. She kept pace with the men the whole length of the parade.

Actor John Travolta's memorable street strut in high-heeled boots in an opening scene of *Saturday Night Fever* beautifully demonstrated how an elevated heel could do as much to add sexiness in masculine movement as in female movement. Not only chic French women know the value of high heels.

MAKING THE EFFORT

French women are willing to put out effort to look attractive. This effort pays big dividends. Yet many American women resent or refuse similar efforts. Two real estate agents showed me the different French and American attitudes.

The condo that I had been leasing was up for sale. The previous day I received a phone call from a local real estate agent who happened to be French. She phoned to make two appointments: the first to preview the condo the next morning, the second to bring a client to view it later that day.

The French real estate arrived the next morning, punctual as well as chic. She wore one the longer skirts in fashion that year, in black of course, paired with a black shirt and a black cardigan-style jacket, dark stockings, and smart black mid-heel pumps. Her jewelry was simple and discreet. A pretty clasp held this French woman's hair artfully on the back of her head. She wore minimal makeup: some foundation, lipstick, but nothing that said makeup, just enough to enhance her natural prettiness. (Her face, hair, eyes and skin tone were much that of Jacqueline Kennedy Onassis.)

Since I know French women's tricks, I soon realized that she was not as slim as I had perceived she was when I first opened the door. Her hips were a tad broad, I realized. But with her lovely straight posture, and by choosing a slimming, neutral color and straight cut in clothing, and by wearing an elevated heel, she put everything nicely in proportion. In total, she was chic, yet appropriately dressed for the warm, humid climate and tendency toward informality of our South Texas city. We discussed the high points and some of the drawbacks to the condo. She thanked me for my time, gave me one of those firm French handshakes, and departed.

That afternoon, the French real estate agent and her client, a man, arrived punctually at the appointed time. The man was clearly pleased to be shown properties by this attractive, well-dressed French woman, with her lovely, modulated voice and its charming accent. It amused me to see her French charm at work. This was, by the way, an excellent example of how French women use their appearance and femininity in a business situation. Yet please understand that she was in not in any way flirtatious. She was behaving in a perfectly professional manner. My guess was, that with the combination of her appearance and her professional approach to selling, her client probably bought one of the several properties she was showing him that day.

The following day, my condo was shown by an American real estate agent. This woman did not preview the property, nor did she phone to make an appointment any reasonable time in advance. She phoned on her cellphone to tell me they were on their way. Her rapid-fire speech was so twangy and nasal it was difficult to understand her.

When I opened the door, I found the real estate agent talking on her cellphone. Her client, a man, was standing next to her looking exasperated. I was soon to realize why.

The real estate agent's lack of professionalism began with her attire. She wore leggings, a rather limp sweat shirt, running shoes and a baseball cap. (I am not making this up. This actually happened *chez moi*.) She was talking on her cellphone when I opened the door, and she continued talking on the cellphone as she entered my condo. The client and I looked at each other. Was this woman going to actually show him the condo? It seemed not; she was unwilling to disconnect herself from her cellphone conversation. So in the interest of time (I wanted to get back to work on this book.) I offered to show the man the condo. The real estate agent remained in my living room the whole time I took her client through the condo. She stood in that hunched, head-down position people often adopt for talking on cellular phones. She was still in conversation on her cellphone as the man thanked me and they left.

The previous day, the French woman's client had given the impression he was greatly enjoying being shown condominiums with beautiful bay views by the attractive, chicly dressed French woman. The client of the American real estate agent seemed embarrassed to be in the company of this sloppily dressed cellphone addict, and apologetic that he had somehow been the cause of bringing her into my home.

I do not know, but I am guessing, that these women likely conduct their personal encounters with men in much the way they approach business matters. The French woman would surely make the effort to be dressed attractively. She would take the time to inform herself of interesting conversation topics to discuss when they were sharing a quiet moment over a glass of wine or a meal. When she was with a man, she would give her full attention to him.

I suspect that this real estate agent who conducted business in clothing more appropriate for amateur softball than real estate might dress for men in personal situations with the same lack of attention to alluring femininity. As for interesting topics of conversation, if she had any, I doubt she ever stopped talking on her cellphone long enough to share them. Giving her full attention to a man she was with does not seem likely.

MYSTIQUE

Part of French women's appeal, particularly their appeal to men, is their mystique. What is mystique? Do you have it? If not, how do you get it? What can having a mystique do for you?

Jacqueline Kennedy Onassis still reigns as the best American example of a woman who practiced the French art of feminine mystique. Though she lived three decades after the assassination of her husband, President John F. Kennedy, she never told us what she felt and thought about being seated next to him during the moments of the fatal shots. She gave few personal interviews over her lifetime, she did not publish her memoirs. Our fascination with this woman never faltered.

Mystique is such a feminine word. We never say a man has mystique. We call him a "man of mystery." In the 1980s, actor Pierce Brosnan gained fame playing the character Remington Steele, a man of mystery with a murky past. Our curiosity about that past was one attraction of Remington Steele, though it trailed the attraction of Mr. Brosnan who portrayed Remington Steele.

The British writer John Fowles wrote in his book *The Aristos*, "When the mystery is gone, the energy is gone." We lose interest when we know the answer. We may be deeply engrossed in the beginning chapters of a mystery novel, but if someone tells us whodunit, our interest in finishing the book shrivels.

If Jackie Onassis is an excellent example of a woman who successfully created her own mystique, author and *Cosmopolitan* magazine editor-in-chief Helen Gurley Brown is an excellent example of a woman who destroys whatever mystique she might have. In her books *Having It All* and *The Late Show*, in chapter after chapter, we learn too much about her. Not only is our interest dulled, but many snippets of information diminish this intelligent and successful woman in our eyes. The less I knew about Helen Gurley Brown, the more I admired her.

Sometimes possessing a mystique has amusing consequences. A close friend, as influenced as I by chic French women, shares minimal information about herself with casual acquaintances. She is well educated, well traveled, and well read. She always has interesting conversation topics in place of personal information.

Several years ago, she became friends with a woman with children about the same age as her own. One day, as the two women sat drinking tea while the children played, the friend said, "Of course people here know that you are an oil heiress." My friend was so startled she almost sloshed her tea in her lap. Words failed her. Her muteness was interpreted as confirmation that she was indeed an oil heiress. She is not.

In most instances, other people can make up much more interesting stories about you than any facts you might supply. The tabloid media makes millions on that very fact. Much of the work creating your mystique will be done by others. All you have to do is find other topics of conversation besides yourself. That's easy. Check out interesting websites. Read books and newspapers. Listen to what interesting, intelligent people have to say. Volunteer for an interesting project.

What are the benefits of a mystique? People, especially men, will find a woman much more interesting if she has not bored them with too many details about herself and her life. The secret is to present yourself as a sufficiently interesting person that people will want to know more. *Please* do not bore others with the facts about your gynecological or menopausal problems.

PARFUM

French women might forsake their beloved high-heels to stroll barefoot on the beach, wear ballerina flats with summer casual, or don boots with jeans, but a chic French women will never abandon her fragrance. Some say she feels improperly dressed without it. Nothing declares a woman's femininity so well as the subtle message communicated by a tantalizing scent.

The French have excelled as *perfumeriers* for centuries. French women are devoted customers of their enchanting products. As part of the establishment of her unique personal style, a French woman will choose one or two signature perfumes. She might try a new one from time to time, but she will always have her signature perfume that best evokes her personal style. Cologne, popular in the USA, is not much used in France. French women find it is too anemic. They prefer the more potent *eau de toilette*. For more intimate occasions, French women generally chose more expensive *parfum*.

The first time I went to buy fragrance at a French *parfumerie*, the chic French woman behind the counter asked me *when* I intended to wear it.

"Quand?"

Seeing I needed a lesson, she explained. For day, an *eau de toilette* would be fine. But for evening, I would need a longer-lasting *parfum*. In that practical and unembarrassed manner that French women have for discussing such subjects, she suggested that I might find myself in an amorous evening during which I would not want my fragrance to fail me. *Quelle horreur!*

Perfume is expensive. But French women believe perfume is well worth the cost. Using perfume gives a woman a feeling of extravagance and luxury, of being cared for. Perfume makes French women feel good about themselves. Feeling good about themselves inspires them to refrain from abusive eating that would damage their health or cause them to gain excess weight.

LINGERIE

Like perfume, French women's lingerie makes them feel pampered and special. And very feminine. What could be more feminine that the smoothness of silk, the caress of satin, the delicacy of fine cotton, the sheerness of lace worn next to the skin as a constant reminder of their womanliness?

In 1998, when France 2 interviewed the head of the French lingerie association and asked why French lingerie sales were up despite the problems in the French economy and the high unemployment, his answer: "French women believe that lingerie is like chocolate, it fights depression." Unlike chocolate, pretty undergarments have no calories.

Lingerie might be useful for shaping the body, but French women use lingerie to shape their mood. On lingerie's role in the lives of French women, Susan Sommers, author of *French Chic*, says, "In fact, for many women, wearing the right underthings—those that help them feel flirty and feminine—may be more important than owning the right skirt or shirt. Beautiful lingerie creates the right mood for the Frenchwoman at every hour of the day and night."

A French woman, describing the feeling of wearing lingerie, said, "It's like a wonderful secret—even if you're the only one who knows it."

Feminine is soft. The soft, delicate nature of the fabric from which fine lingerie is made is a next to the skin reminder of those feminine qualities, even when you are dealing in the harsher worlds of business, politics, academics. French women wear silky lingerie underneath their power suits and their uniforms. Their lingerie keeps them in touch with their femininity.

THE GHOST OF EMILY POST

Many thing that French women do that makes them feminine are the things that, in decades past, were considered in the USA "proper behavior for women." Sometime around 1970, American women decided that "being equal" meant being able to use profanity and to discuss their menstrual problems in mixed company. Proper behavior for women as a concept died about this time.

Proper behavior, as defined in previous days, meant taking small sips and bites. It meant chewing with one's mouth closed. Good manners. By the way, all these "feminine" practices are also techniques that help you eat more slowly, chew more carefully. Good practices that help you feel satisfied with a smaller amount of food. Consequently, you are more likely to be slim.

With their femininity, dressing with allure, speaking in a pleasant voice, cultivating their intellect, acting in a civil manner, by charm, and by lavishing attention on their men, French women achieve satisfying relationships.

GIVE FRENCH MEN SOME CREDIT

French women must not be given all the credit for successful relationships. French men do their part. What exactly do they do? "They make a woman feel like a woman," is the answer you hear. Those famous kisses on the hand. Flirting. Listening to what a woman says. Women thrive on such attentions.

I would add the French male's willingness to bestow gifts is also a nice touch. Though I understand lavishness in gifts has been curtailed by recent difficult economic times Still, it is the thought and gesture that counts. Too, French men are willing to carefully stage a seduction: the quiet dinner in the quaint restaurant, the candlelight, the wine, the music, the whispered words, the touches. Just as French women are practical and realistic about the nature of men, their needs and their limitations, French men are practical about the needs and desires of women. French men seem willing to fulfill those needs and desires.

Dorothy L. Sayers, the British mystery writer who wrote her Lord Peter Wimsey mysteries during the same classic mystery era that Agatha Christie penned her Hercule Poirot whodunits, left an unfinished Lord Peter mystery at her death. *Thrones, Dominations* was completed by Jill Paton Walsh and published in 1998.

A character in *Thrones, Dominations* is a Frenchman, Gaston Chapparelle, an artist painting portraits in London. In a conversation with Lord Peter Wimsey, the artist says that his reputation with women is merely for show. He explains:

> If I painted women in Paris, I would not cause a stir. A Frenchwoman expects to be seriously regarded; it is her due. But your poor cold English beauties, for them it is a thrill to stir the blood that someone looks at them for two seconds together; so I look hard, and I make a few remarks, and soon they are telling me that nobody has ever understood them before as I. It is pitiful, Lord Peter. If they are cold, these English women, it is because they are frozen with neglect.

THE BEST LOVERS

The third Durex Global Sex Survey reported from respondents in 14 countries, that 55 percent said the French were the best lovers. (Perhaps the other 45 percent had simply never had the opportunity to have a love affair with anyone French.)

There might have been some correlation between the survey results and the fact that the French ranked first in frequency of sex with an average of 141 sessions per year (roughly once every two and a half days). For the French, however, a love affair is more than just sex. As much thought and effort goes into the preparation and execution of a romance as into a well-prepared French meal. Actually, well-prepared French meals figure into the planning and execution of a romance.

A love affair begins with flirtation, an hors d'oeuvre, that whets the appetite for more. Just as the French prefer to take time to anticipate and enjoy their meals, they prefer that romance should be anticipated, then a leisurely progress made through its several natural states. Each stage is savored and given the participants' full attention. To the French, the main course, sex, is something exquisite: an art, as cerebral as it is physical. Without the intellectual component, sex would not so enjoyable. Surely that is why French women have endeavored to educate themselves so they have something intelligent to say in every situation, especially intimate ones.

What makes quality of life in France so high is surely that there is an intellectual aspect—not just to sex—but to art, food, architecture, films. No surprise the French are upset about the invasion of American television programs, films and fast food. Few of these can be said to have high intellectual content. Certainly not the fast food.

ETERNAL ADOLESCENCE

American women who have experience with French and other European males find that so many American men seem hopelessly immature, particularly in their sexuality. A revealing portrait of the typical American immature male was played so wonderfully by actor Tim Allen on the successful television show *Home Improvement*. The relationship between husband and wife mirrored those that exist between so many American couples. She is mature. He is immature, vacillating between wanting her to play the role of indulging mother and that of companion/wife. He, who is forever playing with his toys— excuse me, tools—is unwilling to grow up and act in a mature, adult manner.

In one particularly revealing episode, the Tim Allen character complains that he wants more sex in their relationship. When he begins to describe specifically the sort of sexual encounters he wants with his wife, they are the adolescent fantasy version of sex rather than a mature version of sexual relations that acknowledge the particular nature of women's needs and desires.

If the French rank so high in their abilities as lovers, it may be that the men have been willing to grow up and approach sex with mature understanding of women rather than with adolescent fantasy. Immature men cause American women a great deal of frustration. If this frustration causes them to seek out comfort foods, it is surely for some very valid reasons.

FLIRTING

French women have reputations as incessant flirts. But there is a large difference in the style, as well as the objectives, of French (European) and American flirting. In an article on flirting on *Salon.com*, writer Christine Schoefer explained that in the European version, "Flirtation wants nothing except momentary pleasure, it is invigorating, witty, light, even elegant."

In the USA, too often flirting has an objective, it is a strategy in the mating game. This American flirting aims at seduction. It expects results. Sometimes inept flirting is mistaken for sexual harassment. But the distinction between the two is clear. When someone flirts with you, it should make you feel good, desirable. Sexual harassment makes you uncomfortable and sometimes frightened. Flirting is light and playful. Sexual harassment is heavy and demeaning.

In France, for both French men and women, flirting is one of their sensual pleasures. They flirt quite naturally and enjoy it immensely. Their flirting is subtle and makes no immediate demands. Flirting pays a compliment. It is a form of politeness. It has no consequences, just makes you feel good that someone thinks you are sufficiently attractive that they are willing to give you a bit of their time and attention. A moment of flirtation is a shared moment of mutual recognition. It confirms you have done well in creating an alluring personal style.

French flirting thrives on subtlety: glances, gestures, half-smiles. I see the style of flirting in which French women regularly indulge as an acknowledgment of a man's masculinity. It simply sends the message: I find you attractive. That makes men feel good, and they send back reciprocal acknowledgement. Of course, an attractive appearance is helpful to successful and enjoyable flirting. And who would want to overeat and spoil their chances at playing this delicious little game well?

BOUNDARIES

Though French women flirt incessantly, they do so within certain parameters. One does not flirt with strangers on the street, for example. A couple of years ago, an article "Going Solo," by Kristin Hohenadel in *Paris Notes*, laid out the rules very succinctly. She wrote, "French women have perfected the art of unapproachable, icy chic. Always coquettish and pouting, the French woman does not show emotion, and in particular, she does not smile." Kristin Hohenadel warns that American women walking down the street in Paris—and I would add, lots of other places—with a big, wide, open American smiling face will give the impression that they are trying to be picked up. And very likely some man will try.

A well-bred French male would consider it in the poorest of taste to approach a woman without an proper introduction. But France is the most visited country in the world, and there are many men of other nationalities walking around on the streets, as well as con men and pickpockets who prey especially on tourists and women alone.

In France, men on the prowl are called *les dragueurs*, and Kristin Hohenadel outlines basic guidelines for dealing with them. First of all, if a man says "Bonjour," he is not being friendly; he is trying to pick you up. Don't respond. Second, don't meet a man's gaze or look him in the eye. That will be interpreted as encouragement. Keep your eyes downward when you walk. (I would add this is a very good idea in French cities for quite another reason: the plenitude of dog droppings on the sidewalk.)

A savvy friend adds that wearing a great-looking pair of sunglasses is also good protection against meeting a man's gaze as you walk down the street. Sunglasses also allow you more range of vision than keeping your eyes cast downward. I once read that Jacqueline Onassis wore those big sunglasses so that she could look at people, yet they could not see her eyes.

In France you never accept a stranger's invitation to have coffee. Even if he is posing as a visiting professor or some other occupation that sounds totally respectable. Agreeing to having a cup of coffee with a man you meet on the street or in some public place is tantamount to agreeing to sleep with him.

The good news is that it is generally safe for a woman to be out alone in Paris. Just leave your friendly American smile at home, and work on perfecting your unapproachable, icy chic.

STAYING SAFE

In France, to rebuff a man's approach will likely not be met by hostility. French men's egos seem to be in better shape than those of men in many other countries. Still, I have traveled alone all over the world for many years, and though I have found myself in a tight spot on a few occasions, I have always been able to extricate myself unmolested. A useful piece of advice a psychologist friend gave me before I went abroad for the first time in my early twenties. She said, "Never treat a pervert like a pervert. If you put them down or call them names, they feel that they have a right to hurt you because you have insulted them." I have followed her advice and it has kept me unhurt.

Several years ago, I had been doing research in a library all afternoon, and I did not realize it was so late and the downtown area so deserted when I approached the drive-through ATM machine. I had punched in my PIN and was waiting for my cash when I found this rough-looking man standing next to my car door. He was muttering, telling me what he intended to do to me. Some of the things were violent. Some were sexual. Some were an unfortunate combination of both. The next moment, the ATM door raised and there was my cash. I started to grab for it, but a gust of wind whipped through and blew all my money out of the machine and down the driveway behind me.

Any woman with common sense would have abandoned the money, hit the accelerator, and fled. (Exactly what I suggest you do, should you find yourself in a similar situation.) But this was an impecunious period of my life. I was not willing to lose that money. Still there was the man's threats to consider, and I did not relish putting to the test whether this character actually intended to do to me what he said he planned. But I remembered the psychologist's advice. I decided to act if this man were the bank president who had come out to help me pick up my scattered money instead of some stranger making perverted threats.

"Excuse me," I said as I opened the car door and got out.

A wall ran along the bank's driveway, and a curbed bed of shrubs hugged the wall. Every one of my twenty-dollar bills had ended up under a different pyracantha bush. I began collecting the money, making polite conversation as picked up my cash. The man followed along after me and actually extracted two of the twenties from the thorny branches himself. With some ceremony, he presented them to me. I thanked him sincerely, and wished him a good evening.

With all my money retrieved, I got into my car and drove away.

DELUSION IS BLISS

French women tolerate behavior in men for which American women have difficulty showing the same complacency. Yet a study by Sandra Murray, Ph.D., a visiting scholar at the University of Michigan's Institute for Social Research, found that happily married American couples tended to see each other's faults in a positive light. They interpreted these faults as endearing quirks. Over time, "a husband will take on the positive qualities a wife sees in him," Dr. Murray promises us. Somehow, I think those "positive qualities" Dr. Murray promises must develop a little faster in some men than others.

I don't think French women see men's faults as endearing quirks, I think they choose in their own self interest not to criticize those faults or waste any energy trying to change men. These savvy and practical women consistently act in their own best self interest. But they don't kid themselves.

WOMEN OF A CERTAIN AGE

In France, they don't say a middle-aged woman; they say a *"femme d'un certain âge,"* a woman of a certain age. No one need be too certain precisely what that age is.

The French are not so youth focused as Americans. They revere the old—in architecture and in art. The French read the classics; they drive a car long after an American would have traded for a newer model. They keep "as is" their grandmother's furniture, fraying upholstery and all, and their grandfather's apartments, cracks in the walls and worn tile on the floor. When they dine in a restaurant, their focus is on the food, not on the trendiness of the decor.

Note the following quote from Peter Mayle's book *Acquired Tastes,* describing a famous and well-loved Parisian restaurant, *Chez Ami.*

The black-and-white-tiled floor has been worn down in patches to bare concrete. A venerable wood-burning stove squats at one side, its rickety tin flue slung precariously across the ceiling. The walls are the color of roasted leather, black-brown and cracked. Straight-backed wooden chairs, narrow tables with salmon-pink cloths, voluminous napkins plain and serviceable cutlery. No artful lighting, no background music, no bar, no frills. A place to eat."

The French are comfortable with obvious signs of age. The French revere fine old wines. They still prepare many recipes as the master chefs who created them a century or more ago. In France, *la femme mûre,* the "ripe," mature woman too is revered.

Why is it that French women are not penalized as harshly for having lived a number of decades?

Jeannie Rousseau was a French intelligence agent against the Nazis in World War II. She was eventually caught, imprisoned, and tortured near the point of death. In a profile of her, *Washington Post* writer David Ignatius quotes a young male friend of the French woman who said of Jeannie Rousseau's beauty and intelligence at age 78 that she is "the kind of woman who make a man wish he was 25 years older."

French women remain attractive to men when they have reached their fifties, sixties, even eighties. Not only to men of their own age, but men many years their junior.

Why do older French women find themselves more highly valued than older women in many other cultures—particularly the American culture? What encourages them to continue their beauty efforts with the same diligence their entire lives?

French women definitely have better certain age role models. In the USA, too often media attention is on older women whose lives are filled with problems. Other American female celebrities remain in the media focus, yet their plastic surgeries leave their faces looking tighter and tighter and stranger and stranger.

Some American women of a certain age determinedly diet themselves skeletally thin, thinking that their gaunt frames make them look more youthful. Instead, they end up looking, as one American male described them to me, as skeletons with moisturizer.

CONSIDERING FARRAH

A perceptive piece on women aging in the USA and the pitfalls some American women fall into during their "certain age" appeared in one of the Scripps Howard daily publications. The article written by media critic Elaine Liner profiled actress Farrah Fawcett at the time of her fiftieth birthday. In honor of this half-century milestone of the former *Charlie's Angels* star, there had been magazine covers, a promotional video that (though I have not seen the video) I understand showed Farrah smearing her bare breasts and buttocks with paint and slithering across a canvas.

Not really the way most American women celebrate 5-0.

The article began: "She's a sad figure, the 50-year-old bimbo. Frozen in time, she's stuck in the moment when her beauty shown brightest and her personality was its most effervescent." A little further into the story Farrah Fawcett is described as "longlimbed, anorexically thin with a fake-and-bake tan."

The article compares Farrah Fawcett with other 50-ish Hollywood beauties who started out playing ditzes: Susan Sarandon, Goldie Hawn, Diane Keaton, and Sally Field. Elaine Liner writes: "But they evolved, growing beyond the perky gamine stage to become respected actresses who stand for more than testimonials to the endurance of silicone."

All four of those women mentioned above are Oscar winners who have extended their talents. Farrah's Fawcett's greatest achievement to date is given as self-maintenance.

Very appropriately the article quotes the French writer Anaïs Nin on the kind of woman who makes a difficult adjustment to aging. Anaïs Nin says, "She lacks confidence, she craves admiration insatiably. She lives on the reflections of herself in the eyes of others. She does not dare to be herself."

French women dare to be themselves. That is what personal style is all about. And being themselves, they are that self at whatever age they find themselves.

French women have numerous splendid certain age role models. You find these chic, successful, and interesting women in the arts, in government, in business, in education, and in every other area of French life. And the majority of them, even in certain age, are slim.

CERTAIN AGE WITH PIZZAZZ

But no one currently shows us that "certain age" with more pizzazz than Italian-born actress Sophia Loren.

I have long praised Sophia Loren's personal style that takes into account her love of food and her refusal to remake herself to someone else's (skinny) image. I recommended her book *Women & Beauty* designed for the special needs of mature women and written when Sophia Loren had recently turned 50. The May 31, 1999, *People* magazine featured Sophia Loren in a cover story "Sophia Loren Forever Sexy." At nearly 65, she had clearly stolen the show at the Oscars wearing Armani—and her bifocals.

Sophia Loren's beauty secrets revealed in the article are more or less what she recommended in *Women&Beauty*: plenty of rest, including nine or more hours of sleep a night. She rises early. There is a theory, by the way, that every hour of sleep before midnight counts as two. Several women I know who look far younger than their years follow the early-bedtime, early-rising routine. I try.

A second beauty secret: exercise. Sophia Loren has always been a devoted walker. She claims jogging is "too jolting." She does 45 minutes of stretching and abdominal crunches and an hour's walk daily.

Sophia Loren has never been Hollywood's definition of slim. But she has always kept her statuesque figure in balance with healthy eating and exercise. Just as French women do.

French women make the effort to stay chic and slim and to keep their brains active because they know that they will be appreciated by French men—even when they reach that certain age. They make the effort to stay chic and slim and witty and informed so they have something intelligent to say, and keep contention and conflict out of their relationships with men. For that reason, they are enjoyed and appreciated by men of all ages.

What can we say of relationships between men and women in France in comparison with relationships in other parts of the world?

They're better.

Those better relationships between men and women pay off in greater happiness and chicer, slimmer, more attractive bodies for French women. Those better relationships, along with French culture, their art of being women, their chic personal styles, the way they eat and shop and organize their households keep them chic and slim.

My *Chic &Slim* translation of those techniques that keep French women chic and slim can keep you chic and slim too!

GOLDEN RULE OF FRENCH CHIC
KEEP IT SIMPLE

Simple means building your wardrobe around a neutral color such as black, brown, navy, or gray. Adding the "in" color of the season with an accessory.

Simple is tailored, classic clothes with simple lines.

Simple is plain black leather mid-heel pumps.

Simple is having clothes that fit perfectly so you don't have to keep checking if they are gaping open, riding up, pulling out, sagging down or spontaneously performing any rearrangement that will detract from your appearance.

Simple is staying slim so you can make your investment in classic, quality clothes pay off for years and years.

Simple is keeping jewelry to a minimum: your wedding ring or one antique ring, a good watch, earrings in real gold.

Simple is short, perfectly filed nails without colored polish to chip and look tacky.

Simple is an attractive face through healthy eating and drinking and a program of skin care, rather than trying to cover up blemishes with heavy foundations and concealers that can streak and rub off on men's shirts, or gum up your pores.

Simple is a well-cut, low-maintenance, indestructible by wind and rain hairstyle.

Simple is not depending on clothes and accessories to make you look attractive, but rather letting your aura of self-confidence, the way you walk and sit, the intelligent and amusing things you say, the sparkle in your eyes, the tone of your voice, and the alluring fragrance of your perfume make you attractive whether you are wearing a sweater and jeans from the flea market or an evening dress from a famous designer's newest collection.

You Can Too!

How did I make the French system work for me? How can you use *Chic&Slim*, my translation of the French system, to help you live well, eat well, yet still stay slim for the rest of your life? And look very chic in the process?

First of all, you must believe in your success.

Chic&Slim techniques cannot help you if you allow negativity to block your success. I *always* believed that someday, somehow, I would lose my fat. My childhood, adolescence, and young adult years can be summed up in two words: fat and miserable. I truly cannot remember a time in my early years when my chubby thighs did not rub together and when my butterball of a body did not fall behind panting with a pain in my side whenever I tried to run and play with other children.

When I was six the family doctor put me on diet pills. "These will take care of her appetite," I remember him confidently telling my mother as he wrote the prescription for amphetamines (amphetamines I later read were taken off the market by the FDA). In any case, the pills did nothing to curb *my* appetite.

Other diets followed. Some diets were prescribed by doctors, some were found in magazines, others were shared by friends. Like so many other fatties, I would struggle and struggle to lose 10 or 15 pounds, (once even 20!!), then I would gain back what I lost. And more. What a waste of effort. Or was it?

A psychologist I knew always said that nothing you do in your life is ever wasted. He believed that even your traumas and your mistakes ultimately were useful to you. If nothing else, if you did something so totally dumb that you regretted it the rest of your life, you were reasonably sure that you would not be tempted to do such a stupid thing again.

Years of failed diets achieved no permanent weight loss, yet I did learn much that was useful to me later when I discovered chic French women's *art de maigrir,* art of slimming.

For me, those early diets were like learning to play scales in your first years of studying a musical instrument.

One thing I learned from traditional diets was calorie content of foods. I don't count calories anymore. Nor do I think that you are more likely to have a successful weight loss if you do count. Chic and slim French women certainly do not count calories or fat grams. Yet because of my early calorie-counting diets, I have a general idea of how many calories in foods I eat. I try to keep eating high-calorie, high-fat foods in healthy moderation. Yet I surprise myself with really how many more calories a day I eat than the maximum recommended for someone my height and body build. But I learned from French women it is not only *what* foods you eat. *How* and *when* you eat and in what *mood* are also important. Personal style plays a major role too.

TINY WOMEN EATING LIKE PIGS

A woman who bought *Chic&Slim* in the Garden District Book Shop in New Orleans said, "I've just spent two weeks in France. In all the restaurants, I saw those tiny French women eating like pigs. I want to know how they do it."

The original *Chic&Slim* began the explanation. *Chic&Slim Encore* was written to give you more French tricks for eating rich food and staying slim and to answer questions that you have asked.

Today in the USA, negativity complicates successful weight loss. Result of what I call *Le Nouveau Puritanisme*. Chic French women are not puritanical. Chic French women do not believe staying slim requires discomfort and deprivation. The French system makes eating well and staying slim a pleasure.

Even if you survive the onslaught of puritanical negativity, your weight loss efforts can be sabotaged by jealous individuals. As Professor of Law and television commentator Susan Estrich writes in her book *Making the Case for Yourself: A Diet Book For Smart Women.*

They need you to fail, not because they hate you, but because that way, they won't have to give up donuts. Some of the thin ones don't want you to get thin, because then it will matter more to them that you're smarter, or prettier, or have blonder hair. They like being the thin one. For some, it's all they have.

The diet failure rate in the USA is high. Frankly, I think that many people fail on diets and in weight control programs simply because, deep in their hearts, they really do not want to be slim. Dieting or paying money for a weight control program enables them to say, "I'm *trying* to do something about my weight."

A mental block to weight loss was never my problem. I sincerely wanted to lose weight. And as soon as I found a workable system that fit my personality, I did lose weight. A film I saw when I was about 10 convinced me the French had answers to my problem.

IT ALL STARTED WITH SABRINA

Many of us can look back to a film or a book that made a difference in our lives. For me, the film was the 1954 movie *Sabrina*, the version starring Audrey Hepburn in the title role. Sabrina, the awkward and insecure chauffeur's daughter, is sent to Paris to cooking school. She returns sophisticated, not just in her appearance—though in Givenchy she looked stunning—she is also worldly, confident, and in control of life. And she knows how to handle men.

In a scene in which Sabrina preparing to return to the USA writes to her father, she tells him she has learned so much more than how to prepare French cuisine. "I have learned many more important things. I have learned how to live. How to be *in* the world, and *of* the world. And not just to stand aside and watch."

In our first view of Sabrina on her return from Paris we see her standing in the Glen Cove train station, wearing that figure-hugging Givenchy suit and hat, with her French poodle on a leash. Her outfit screams French chic. That Audrey Hepburn, the epitome of slimness, played Sabrina sent its own message. I walked out of the movie theater convinced that, from the French, I could learn not only how to be slim, but I would learn something more: *savoir-vivre*, how to live.

FURTHER INSPIRATION

If I had any remaining doubts that the French might offer improvement for my life, in the early 1960s, two American women convinced me. First Lady Jacqueline Kennedy became a role model. As I read and reread her biography and countless media stories about her, I came to believe that what molded Jacqueline Kennedy into a woman who would intrigue and inspire millions was the time she had spent in France. As France had transformed the fictional Sabrina, France had transformed young Jacqueline Lee Bouvier into a uniquely elegant and successful female.

President and Mrs. Kennedy installed a French chef and a French pastry chef in the White House. In the early 1960s, those of us not receiving invitations to dine at the Executive Mansion were discovering the joys of French cuisine, thanks to the efforts of another American woman, Julia Child. As a college student on a limited budget, I could not afford her *Mastering the Art of French Cooking*. I had to settle for one of the many French cookbooks in English the popularity of *Mastering* spawned.

My humble substitute was a decent little cookbook. Paperback, of course. The first lesson I learned about French cooking was that the French waste nothing. Later, when I had more first-hand knowledge of French cuisine, I sometimes cynically thought that the reason the

French stayed so slim was that some of their dishes certainly did not encourage second helpings. (Some, as far as I'm concerned, did not encourage first helpings.) In fact, some French delicacies are prepared from things that Americans don't want discussed at the table, much less served on their plates.

FRENCH LESSONS

My instinct as a 10-year-old in the movie theater watching *Sabrina* was correct: the French could teach me lessons that would bring positive changes. When I returned to the small town in Oklahoma town where I had grown up, I might not have looked like Audrey Hepburn wearing Givenchy, but I looked better. I was certainly slimmer than when I had left.

Chic&Slim, my translation of the French system, is based on techniques I learned from French women. It does contain some deviations from how the French live and eat in France. To stay slim outside France requires modifying the basic French system.

Chic&Slim Encore gives you more of what I have learned in my decades of successfully staying slim. I have kept the Fat Monster at bay through marriage, motherhood, divorce, major illness, financial hardship, and the glories of that "certain age." This book is designed to give you the techniques and tools for a lifestyle that can make you slim, happy, and successful. And chic. *Certainement* chic!

You have read the theory. The following sections of *Chic&Slim Encore* are devoted to resources to help you lose weight and stay slim *à la Anne Barone*. First are portion guidelines and menus. Next come 20 favorite recipes, dishes I eat on a regular basis to keep me healthy and slim.

A fatty like me lost 55 pounds and I stay slim using this French-inspired *Chic&Slim* system. **You Can Too!**

UNDERSTATED FRENCH INSOUCIANCE

The coup de grace is that she made it look as if she wasn't trying too hard. That, of course, is the elusive essence of "understated" French insouciance—the thing that only gets better in amazing Parisian middle-age.

Sarah Mower, Fashion Writer

THANKS FOR CHIC & SLIM

Bonjour Anne!

Thank you so much for the fast delivery of the Chic and Slim books. I just love them. It is so good to hear I can eat bread, and with butter, no less. Brought my bread machine up from the basement and made some yesterday. I am actually cooking again, instead of buying whatever frozen low fat dinners are on sale that week. Living alone, I had fallen into bad habits, like eating standing up at the counter. Now I sit down and use real dishes and trying out new wines. Such a more civilized way to live.

I have been reading the website, it's great. Thanks for all you are doing. Heaven knows Americans need it!

Au revoir! — *Sandy in MA*

YOUNGER THAN THEIR AGE

Fat people often appear younger than their chronological age. The skin doesn't seem to age so quickly. While I don't think anyone would recommend overweight, there's no question an older woman looks better with a *little* extra weight.

Diane von Furstenberg, Fashion Designer

7

PORTIONS & MENUS

THE *Chic&Slim* PHILOSOPHY BELIEVES EVERY WOMAN is unique. That every woman has a different body, lifestyle, personal style, activity level, age, and health. How much food and what foods she must eat to lose weight and stay slim are unique to her.

If you are a 22-year-old, five-foot-ten woman who plays racquetball one hour, five days a week, you would be miserably hungry restricting yourself to a menu that would maintain a normal, healthy weight in a 52-year-old, five-foot-two woman who took a brisk, 30-minute walk each day.

Dictating what foods and how much to eat of those foods are what diets do. Diets don't work.

For that reason, in the original *Chic&Slim* book there were no dictated portion sizes and no suggested menus. Experience with the French system taught me that to stay slim, it is not *what* you eat, but *how* you eat that is most important. Recent medical research has confirmed my personal findings.

When I returned to live in the United States, I went through a phase in which I ate a great deal of American fast food and convenience food. Finally, one day my son announced that if I served pizza one more time, he was going to start eating supper at his grandmother's.

Still, during my American fast food and convenience food phase, I stayed slim. I might have been eating burgers, pizzas, and fried chicken, but I was using techniques that keep the French slim: eating slowly, moderate portions, sitting at a table to eat, no snacking between meals, keeping refined sugar in my diet minimal, eating plenty of fresh vegetables and fruit, and doing regular exercise.

So I believed that not only were portion guidelines and menus unnecessary, but they might be counterproductive.

Then, I received an email from a *Chic&Slim* reader who wrote:

Would you ever consider posting a "sample menu" of a typical day's eats for you? I know that a specific menu contradicts the general style changes you endorse, but so many of us are so far gone, so inundated with lousy eating info (info that our chubby friends, co-workers, and families reinforce) that we honestly aren't always sure what's really constitutes "eating right." Is a good breakfast, ONE slice of bread or two? How many nibbles of pâté can we safely afford? Once we get the general gist of it, we can do it on our own.

She made a convincing argument. I reminded myself that I had the advantage that I had observed French women at their own tables. Yet many who read the *Chic&Slim* books and website information on *annebarone.com* have not had the same opportunity to observe chic French women. I relented.

The following portion size and menu guidelines are given with the caveat that ultimately only *you* (with the advice and counsel of your health care professional) can decide what and how much you can eat and stay slim.

CHIC & SLIM PORTIONS

Meat, fish, poultry—3 1/2 ounces cooked

Raw vegetables—1 cup

Cooked vegetables—1/2 cup

Sorbet or mousse—1/3 cup

Yogurt—1/2 cup

Fresh fruit—1 medium

Chopped fresh fruit—1/2 cup

Bread—1 slice

Baguette—3 inch piece

Soup—1 cup

Pasta or Rice or Noodles—1/2 cup cooked

Hard or semi-soft cheese—1 ounce

How much meat is 3 1/2 ounces (100 grams)? A boneless portion about the size of the plastic case for a cassette audiotape. Remember cassettes? Perhaps it is easier to think in terms of the size of most pressed powder compacts.

One ounce of cheese measures about 1 inch (2 1/2 cm.) square. But chic French women would probably eat only half that amount in the cheese course of a meal. By one cup, I mean the standard dry measure —or liquid measure of 8 fluid ounces.

While you adjust to chic French portions, it is useful to actually measure your portions with standardized measuring containers until your eye learns to judge accurately. Soon it becomes automatic.

The most successful strategy for cutting back on the amount of food you eat is to reduce portion sizes gradually. I repeat, gradually.

CHIC & SLIM STRATEGY
REDUCING PORTION SIZES

Gradual portion size reduction is the success secret.

If you are a between-meal snacker, do not attempt to give up *all* your between-meal snacks at once. Cut back on the amount you eat at one snack. After you have adjusted comfortably to that, eliminate that snack. Repeat the process with another between-meal snack. Finally, work toward eliminating before-bedtime snacking. (Note: I do not consider afternoon tea a snack. Afternoon tea is a sanity restorer and recharger. Afternoon tea is therapy.)

Before you begin making major changes in what foods you eat on a regular basis, try cutting back on portion sizes of your usual foods. One helping instead of two. Instead of eight ounces of meat and one-half cup of cooked vegetables, try five ounces of meat and one cup of cooked vegetables. You may not need to learn to cook new dishes. Simply *stop overeating* the dishes you like and enjoy.

Do not eat food for which you have no real hunger. That means you don't eat that sandwich on your toddler's plate just because it's there. And we have all been at someone's home, and there is food left in the serving dish, and the hostess shoves the dish toward us and says, "Here, you finish this."

"And who appointed me the designated garbage disposal for this evening?" I have to bite my tongue to keep from asking.

Say no-thank-you to food for which you have no hunger, and especially to food you do not really like. Be alert to food pushers who try to pressure you to eat more food than you want or need. Trying to force a guest to overeat is not hospitality. It is bad manners.

And remember your stomach is about the same size as your fist. Keep your food intake in proportion to your stomach size.

CHIC & SLIM MENUS

BREAKFAST

Breakfast is my favorite meal of the day. If I thought I had to launch my day with yogurt, fresh fruit, and herbal tea as so many weight-loss diets recommend, I probably wouldn't bother to get out of bed. I certainly would not get out of bed to eat dry cereal!

For breakfast I want good bread. I need caffeine.

Breakfast for me must be a standard French breakfast: coffee or hot tea with good fresh bread spread with a little butter and all-fruit jam. The French call bread spread with butter and jam a *tartine*. If I am feeling especially hungry, I will add a hard-boiled egg or one-half cup plain yogurt, perhaps with a tablespoon of brewer's yeast stirred into the yogurt. Sometimes I substitute flaxseed oil for butter.

Mornings that I am at the computer before 6 AM, I may eat a small *tartine* with early tea, then, a proper breakfast mid-morning. If I have gained a few pounds, then, on rising I drink a cup of warm water with a squeeze of lemon juice, then have my usual French breakfast later. In weight loss mode, I might skip jam and eat only butter or flaxseed oil with my bread. I will drink my coffee or hot tea without milk. Whole grain breads make a heartier breakfast that will keep me feeling full and satisfied longer than an white flour French baguette. Whole grain bagels made without fats and sugars also make a good *Chic&Slim* breakfast bread.

Café au lait: 4 fluid ounces strong hot French roast coffee mixed with four fluid ounces hot milk.

Tea: As a dedicated tea lover, I generally prefer loose teas. But for breakfast tea these days, I choose the convenience of tea bags, pyramids or cushions. Assams are hearty breakfast teas. Ceylons more delicate.

Tartine: 4-inch length French bread (baguette 3 inches diameter) spread with 1/4 teaspoon unsalted butter + 2 teaspoons all-fruit jam.

LIGHTER MEAL OF THE DAY

In the past, many slim French women ate their more substantial meal mid-day. Two-hour lunch hours made that possible. Now in France, as in the USA, most women who work simply do not have the time to eat their largest meal mid-day. They must make do with a light lunch and eat the larger meal in the evening. When I was losing my excess weight, I was eating a lighter lunch and often eating four and five-course meals fashionably late in the evening. From my experience, what really matters is the total amount of food you eat in any 24-hour period. Some weight control experts disagree with my experience.

Rather than call these menus Lunch and Dinner, I call them Lighter Meal of the Day and More Substantial Meal of the Day. Plug them into the clock at whatever time suits your lifestyle.

A symbol (❧) before the menu item indicates the recipe is included in the recipe section of this book.

❧ French Lentil Soup
Slice Sourdough Bread

——— ——— ——— ——— ———

Cheese Omelette   Brussels Sprouts
❧ Baguette   Pear with Goat Cheese

——— ——— ——— ——— ———

Plate of Crudities (raw, low-cal veggies)
❧ Maria's *Migas*   1 Orange or 1/2 Grapefruit

——— ——— ——— ——— ———

❧ *Ratatouille*
❧ Baguette   Cherries, Fresh or Frozen

——— ——— ——— ——— ———

❧ The Ambassador's *Borscht*
Whole Grain Rye Roll

—— — — — — —

✤ *Galettes* with steamed spinach topped with poached egg
Apple

—— — — — — —

✤ *Pan Bagnat*
Melon Wedge

AFTERNOON TEA

—— Ceylon Tea
Applesauce Raisin Muffin

—— Darjeeling Tea
Cucumber Sandwich

—— Taylors of Harrogate Yorkshire Gold Tea
Scone

—— Assam Tea
✤ Certain Age Cheesecake with Blueberries

—— Earl Grey Tea
1 Fig Bar

—— Coffee
1 Small Mexican Pastry with Sliced Kiwi

—— Jasmine Green Tea
✤ 1 *Sablé* and 2 Fresh Strawberries

MORE SUBSTANTIAL MEAL

⚜ *Poulet en Cocotte Barone*

⚜ Rice or Millet   Lemon Tart

—   —   —

Salmon with Fresh Dill and Lemon Juice

Steamed Broccoli

⚜ Baguette   French Flan

—   —   —

⚜ *Couscous*

Fresh Apricots and California Dates

—   —   —

⚜ Phil's Squash   Green Beans

Salad (Curly Red Leaf with Oil and Vinegar)

Apples Baked in Molasses and Butter

—   —   —

⚜ *Viande Rouge Jacques*   ⚜ Brown Rice

Mousse au Chocolat

—   —   —

Fish, Baked with Lemon Juice and Olive Oil

⚜ *Tabouli*   Zucchini

—   —   —

Grilled Lean Beef OR Chicken Thigh OR Grilled Slice of Tofu

Potatoes Roasted in Olive Oil and Rosemary

Red Cabbage with Apples   Fruit Compote

Chic & Slim Recipes

Delicious recipes from all over the world

For decades, living and traveling all over the world, I have collected recipes for delicious, healthy food. My weekly menu might have been planned by committee at the United Nations. Of course, my menus contain many delicious French dishes. French breads and pastries, classic French onion soup, favorite Riviera beach food, a vegetable casserole from Provence, and dozens more. All are served often.

Tailored to keep you healthy and slim

Like many cooks, I make modifications to recipes I collect. Through the years these recipes have evolved to incorporate availability of ingredients, my own taste preferences, and some of the latest nutritional research about what foods make and keep us healthy and slim.

Fast and easy preparation

I love good food. But I do *not* like to cook. I hate cleanup. You will find I have streamlined these recipes to be as quick and easy as possible without compromising nutrition and taste.

Good for women. Delicious to all.

Like many women of a "certain age," I am trying to eat more soy. Okay, so tofu tastes like congealed latex paint and textured soy protein has all the exciting flavor and aroma of foam rubber pellets. But blended into a fruit-garnished cheesecake this healthy low-cost food can be quite delicious.

As sweet as need be

One of the best slimming lessons I learned from the French was the importance of keeping the amount of refined sugar eaten to a minimum. My goal is always to eat NO refined sugar, nor any foods that contain any of the alternate forms: dextrose, fructose, and all those other names that the food industry likes to put on the label to keep you from realizing how much sugar they are adding to their products. Of course *never* eating any refined sugar is impossible. But since I do not eat processed pseudo-foods, sugar avoidance is much easier. That does not mean skipping desserts and pastries, however. Though the years I have reprogrammed my taste buds so that they find "sweet" foods that contain less refined sugar than those I ate as a fatty.

If you are accustomed to eating American desserts made by traditional recipes, or if you regularly eat commercially made cookies, cakes, and pies, you will probably find that, at first, the cheesecake and the cookies in this recipe section are not sweet enough for you. You can simply add sugar to the recipe, or you can sprinkle on some honey or other sweetener before serving.

As far as weight control and your general health goes, one of the best favors you can do yourself is to keep the amount of refined sugar in your diet limited. Just as the French do.

CALORIES AND FAT GRAMS

How many calories and fat grams are in these recipes?

I have no idea. Chic French women do not tally calories and fat grams. Neither do I. My diet is good, well-prepared food, moderate portions, chewing slowly and carefully. If my jeans begin feeling tight, I cut back on the amount of bread I eat and increase the amount of low-calorie veggies. I make an effort to increase the number of times a week I exercise.

I eat for taste and pleasure and for keeping my body healthy. When I make sure that I eat healthy food, then, I am not hungry for snacks and *junque* food that put on extra pounds. It's that simple.

Now the recipes. *Bon appétit!*

Chic & Slim Recipes

French Bread (Machine Version)
Pain aux Céréales
Galettes (Buckwheat Crêpes)
Ratatouille Barone
Phil's Squash
Salade Niçoise
Anne Barone's Tabouli
The Ambassador's Borscht
French Onion Soup
Poulet en Cocotte Barone
French Lentil Soup
Viande Rouge Jacques
Brown Rice
Pan Bagnat (Sandwich)
Maria's Migas (Egg & Vegetable Dish)
Couscous
Certain Age Cheesecake
Sablés
Chic&Slim Jam

Key to Abbreviations
tsp. = teaspoon   Tbs. = tablespoon
oz. = ounce   lb. = pound
in. = inch   med. = medium   F. = Fahrenheit

FRENCH BREAD
(BREAD MACHINE VERSION)

Most French bread sold in the United States resembles real French bread to about the same extent that most American women resemble French actresses Audrey Tautou or Catherine Deneuve. So how do you find good French-style bread in the USA? You bake it.

I make a good French-style baguette allowing my 2 lb. capacity bread maker to mix, knead, and do the first rising. Then I shape the baguettes by hand before the second rising. You can make the recipe using all unbleached flour, or half unbleached and half whole wheat. French bread by law is flour, water, salt, yeast. Despite that many American "French" bread recipes call for it, sugar is not necessary to activate the yeast. I have made bread for years without a granule of sugar.

INGREDIENTS:

4 1/3 cups wheat flour	1 3/4 cups water
3 tsp. "instant" yeast	2 tsp. salt

White cornmeal to sprinkle on baking sheet.

METHOD:

Follow the machine's instructions for the order in which the ingredients are placed in mixing pan. Use the water temperature your machine's instructions specify. When the machine signals dough is ready, remove from the pan. Sprinkle a bread board, or clean, dry, work surface, lightly with flour. Divide dough into three portions. If you aren't familiar with shaping baguettes, consult a cookbook. Julia Child's cookbooks are the definitive word on French bread making. Shape dough into three baguettes. Arrange on a baking sheet sprinkled with white cornmeal, or a perforated baguette pan. Set the baguettes in a warm place and allow dough to rise until double in bulk. (Approximately 1 hour.) Preheat oven to 425 degrees F. Bake baguettes for 15 minutes at 425 degrees F. Lower the temperature to 400 degree F. and bake an additional 10 minutes. Turn off the oven and allow the baguettes to remain in the oven for 10 more minutes to make the crust really wonderful.

PAIN AUX CÉRÉALES
(GRAINS BREAD)

Pain aux Céréales is the popular bread in France these days. Far tastier and more nutritious than the traditional baguette, this grains bread is very popular with chic and slim French women. Especially those women wishing to shed a kilo or two. My version of *pain aux céréales*, made easily in a bread machine, is inspired by the Paris favorite grains bread, that baked by master French baker Eric Kayser at his Maison Kayser. You can eat this grains bread with cheese, spread it with pâté, in a sandwich, or toasted with jam. Eat it the day you bake it. Or slice and freeze. Look in the natural foods section of your supermarket for hulled millet, sesame and sunflower seeds. Warning: This bread is so good, it is almost addictive.

INGREDIENTS:

2 Tbs. hulled millet	1 1/2 cups water
3 cups unbleached flour	1/4 cup sunflower seeds
3/4 cup rolled oats	1 tsp. sea salt
1 Tbs. sesame seed	2 1/4 tsp. "instant" yeast
1 Tbs. sesame seed for crust	

METHOD: Place the millet in the bottom of the bread machine's baking pan. Pour in the water, then add the flour, rolled oats, sesame and sunflower seeds and salt. Make a well in the center of the flour and place the yeast. Set the machine for the 3-hour Normal bake cycle. Set a kitchen timer for 1 hour 5 minutes. When the timer rings, check to see that the last kneading is finished (approximately 1 hour 55 minutes before finish). Before bread dough begins to rise again, sprinkle 1 Tbs. sesame seed over the top and sides of dough. The seeds will bake into the crust. The crunchy, delicious taste these outer seeds give to the crust is worth the extra effort to add the second tablespoon of sesame seeds after the last kneading.

GALETTES

Galettes are a favorite French street food. The French like to eat these paper-thin buckwheat crêpes folded over a fried egg and spinach—and sometimes a bit of ham. Americans in France like *galettes* for breakfast spread with some good French butter and jam, or drizzled with honey. For a successful *galette*, you must have a thin batter and tilt the hot griddle quickly so that the batter will spread well. *Galette* batter must be mixed ahead of time, at least an hour, and best left in the refrigerator overnight and then taken out an hour before cooking.

INGREDIENTS:

2 eggs

1 cup milk   1 cup water

1 Tbs. canola oil

1 cup buckwheat flour   1/2 tsp. salt

1/2 cup unbleached wheat flour

Additional canola oil for cooking

METHOD: Whisk the eggs in a batter bowl with the milk, water, and canola oil. Stir in the flours and salt until well blended. Batter should be like thin cream. If not, add more milk. Cover and let the batter sit at room temperature for 1 hour, or overnight in refrigerator. Remove from refrigerator at least an hour before cooking.

To cook, heat a 10-inch non-stick griddle or skillet until hot enough that a drop of water sizzles on the cooking surface. Brush with a little oil. Flours settle. Stir batter before cooking each *galette*. Pour approximately 1/4 cup batter onto griddle and tilt quickly to cover the cooking surface. Cook *galette* 1 minute. Turn and cook 30 seconds on other side. Stack cooked *galettes* on a plate. Reheat when serving.

Galettes, once cooled, can be separated with waxed paper and placed in an air-tight plastic bag and stored in the refrigerator 1-2 days or frozen for later use for eating both savory and sweet.

RATATOUILLE BARONE

Ah, summer in the south of France! You would be sure to enjoy the region's wonderful vegetables. This vegetable casserole tastes of Mediterranean sunshine with flavors of tomatoes, eggplant, onions, garlic, shiny zucchini all baked in green-gold olive oil and flavored with tangy fresh herbs. One of my favorite dishes and a staple of my summer eating. Resist the temptation to top it with cheese. The olive oil flavor is too exquisite to mask with dairy. Serve with grilled chicken or fish. Or eat with crusty French bread and a salad for a light summer meal. Red wine or chilled mineral water with lemon for your beverage.

INGREDIENTS:

4 zucchini, 6 to 8 inches, sliced into coins

2 yellow onions, sliced medium thin

1 large eggplant, peeled and cubed

8 Roma (plum) tomatoes, quartered

8 cloves garlic, peeled   1/4 tsp. dried thyme

1/4 cup fresh basil leaves   1/4 cup olive oil

salt and pepper to taste.

METHOD; Preheat oven to 300 degrees F. Layer vegetables and herbs in a large oven-safe casserole. Pour olive oil over vegetables and cover. Bake covered for 2 1/2 to 3 hours.

PHIL'S SQUASH

Here is my favorite way to prepare butternut squash. Years ago, Uncle Phil had a bumper crop of butternut squash on his Pennsylvania farm. At a family dinner, he served his special way of preparing this tasty vegetable. Every fall at the peak of the season, I prepare this dish several times made with organic butternut squash from Colorado. With a salad and some hearty bread, this dish makes a light supper. For a more substantial meal, pair it with roast chicken or pork chops.

INGREDIENTS Phil's Squash:

 1 medium butternut squash, peeled and cubed

 2 Tbs. butter *or* canola oil

 1/4 lb. grated cheese, mozzarella or cheddar

 1/2 tsp. salt

 Course ground black pepper to taste

 Method: Peel and seed the squash and cut into 1 inch cubes. In a non-stick pan heat butter to bubbly over medium heat. Sauté squash cubes about 10 minutes, turning when needed. Cover and cook over low heat until squash is tender. If squash becomes too dry during cooking, add a small amount of water to prevent sticking. When squash is tender, sprinkle with salt and stir in the cheese. Garnish with black pepper.

SALADE NIÇOISE

Salade Niçoise is the perfect chic French Riviera salad for those lazy hot days at the beach or by the pool. Everyone has their own version. Mine always includes tuna. But I often skip the anchovies. Traditionally, you neither toss nor add dressing to *Salade Niçoise*. You can place cruets of olive oil and vinegar on the table for those who want more dressing.

INGREDIENTS:

 1 head Boston or Romaine lettuce, washed and torn

 1 5-oz can albacore tuna   1 Tbs. olive oil   2 tsp. vinegar

 1/2 lb. green beans, steamed

 5 medium tomatoes, peeled, seeded, and quartered

 1 red or green pepper, in thin circles   1 Tbs. capers

 1 small cucumber, peeled and thinly sliced

 4 hard-cooked eggs, quartered   1/4 cup parsley leaves

 10 stuffed green olives, halved   15 basil leaves

 1 2-oz. can flat anchovy fillets (optional)

METHOD: Steam the green beans 10 minutes. While beans are hot, toss with the olive oil and vinegar. If using water-packed tuna, drain and sprinkle with 1 to 2 Tablespoons olive oil. Arrange the lettuce on a large serving plate. Flake the tuna over the lettuce. Layer the rest of the ingredients in the following order: tomatoes, green beans, pepper rings, cucumber, hard-cooked eggs, anchovy fillets, olives, basil, parsley, capers.

In the classic *The Food of France*, author Waverly Root tells us that the food of Nice is outdoor food. This most famous salad of Nice tastes best outdoors. A chilled mineral water is a great accompaniment.

ANNE BARONE'S TABOULI

The secret to the flavor of this summer salad is the harmony in the quartet of flavors. Full, mellow olive oil. Tangy lemon. Clean, crisp mint. Spicy onion. Usually made with bulgur, my version uses brown rice. Also delicious when quinoa replaces the bulgur. This salad goes well with almost anything that comes off the grill. Or you can eat the salad as a light lunch or supper. Chilled melon makes a great way to end the meal.

INGREDIENTS:

4 cups cooked brown rice or quinoa   3 Tbs. olive oil

1 cup chopped fresh mint leaves

2 bunches parsley, finely chopped (flat Italian is best)

1 cucumber, peeled and sliced   5 green onions, thinly sliced

Juice of 1 large or 2 small lemons   1/8 tsp. black pepper

3/4 tsp. salt, preferably sea salt

METHOD: Combine ingredients in a large bowl, mix well, cover, and chill in the refrigerator 1 to 6 hours to allow the flavors to blend. Serve tabouli over a bed of crisp Romaine leaves.

THE AMBASSADOR'S BORSCHT

When I served in the United States Peace Corps in West Africa in the 1960s, the American Ambassador's cook made this wonderful cold beet soup that was often served as a first course at luncheons at the Ambassador's residence. Delicious in hot weather. *Crème fraîche* figured in the Ambassador's cook's version. Back in the USA, when I couldn't buy *crème fraîche*, I used sour cream. A friend, whose family had immigrated to the USA from Russia, made a similar soup in which she used cultured buttermilk. Such a reduction in calories from sour cream. Almost every brand of buttermilk I find these days has additives I don't like. I have settled on using plain yogurt. Non-fat yogurt works well. Low-fat tastes better. Whole milk yogurt is wonderful.

INGREDIENTS:

3-4 medium fresh beets, peeled and sliced

(or 1 15-oz. can sliced beets)

1 yellow onion, peeled and quartered

4 stalks celery, cut in 3 in. lengths

2 medium carrots, cut in 1 in. lengths

5 cloves of garlic, peeled

2 cups beef or vegetable broth

2 cups water (*or* 1 cup water if using canned beets)

Plain yogurt   1 lemon

METHOD: In a large saucepan combine all ingredients except yogurt and lemon. Use beet liquid as well as beets if using canned. Bring to boil. Lower heat and simmer until vegetables test tender with a fork. Cool slightly. Put vegetables and liquid into blender or food processor. Puree. Chill the vegetable puree in the refrigerator until time to serve.

To serve: Mix two parts vegetable puree to one part yogurt. Squeeze in juice of one-eighth lemon for each one-cup serving. Garnish with a slice of fresh lemon. A great hot weather soup.

FRENCH ONION SOUP

A cool rainy evening, a simmering pot of French onion soup, a bottle of red wine, some French cheese and a crusty baguette. Give me those and I think I am in Paris. My version of French onion soup uses chopped instead of the more usual sliced onions. Chopped onions cook more quickly and make a soup that is easier to eat chicly. The chic French women I knew always made onion soup with bouillon cubes. Bouillon cubes today are mostly salt, so if you have no homemade, use a commercial beef broth such as Pacific or a "beef base" if your budget is tight. Read the label to make sure you aren't just getting salt, sugar, and chemicals—and no beef. Buy imported Gruyère cheese. Much American swiss-style cheese has such high moisture content that it is not really less expensive. Also flavor is sometimes lacking.

INGREDIENTS:

1/3 cup olive oil

4 medium yellow onions, peeled and chopped

4 cloves garlic, peeled and minced

1 quart. beef broth

   (or 4 tsp. beef base dissolved in 1 quart hot water)

1/4 tsp. dried sage   1 bay leaf   2 sprigs fresh thyme

Gruyère cheese

METHOD:

Heat the oil in a heavy-bottomed saucepan, add onions. Cook over high heat 5-7 minutes, stirring to prevent sticking. Lower heat to medium hot and continue to cook the onions 30 to 35 minutes, stirring when needed to prevent sticking. Turn off the heat and stir in the minced garlic. Add the beef broth, sage, bay leaf, and thyme. Bring to boil. Immediately lower heat and simmer for 30 minutes. To serve, remove bay leaf and thyme sprig and ladle into warmed bowls. Top with a generous amount of grated *Gruyère*. Croutons? *Si vous voulez.*

POULET EN COCOTTE BARONE

This recipe for a whole chicken roasted in a casserole (*en cocotte*) and the following recipe for French Lentil Soup are good examples of how chic French women plan menus so that one night's dinner becomes the basis for the next night's. The lentil soup recipe will use the *restes*, leftovers from this roast chicken and vegetables.

INGREDIENTS:

1 whole chicken (2 1/2 - 3 1/2 pounds)

6 carrots, peeled and cut in thirds

8 celery stalks, cut in fourths

4 onions, cut in fourths   4 turnips, peeled and quartered

6 cloves of garlic, peeled   2 Tbs. olive oil

4 sprigs thyme   salt and pepper to taste

METHOD:

Preheat the oven to 400 degrees F. Prepare the vegetables and arrange in a ovenproof casserole dish large enough for the chicken plus all the vegetables. Put the chicken on top the vegetables and brush the chicken with the olive oil. Arrange 3 thyme sprigs on chicken and tuck one in the cavity. Cover with lid or aluminum foil. Bake 1 hour. Remove the covering and baste chicken and vegetables with cooking juices. Continue to roast chicken for about another hour, basting with cooking juices at 20 minute intervals until chicken is golden brown and cooking thermometer registers 165 degrees F. After the meal, refrigerate the remaining chicken, vegetables and cooking juices for making soup the following day. It is time-saving if you can roast the chicken and vegetables in a casserole dish that is also suitable for storing the left-overs in the refrigerator.

A French woman is always sure how much her family will eat at any time. She can calculate the exact amount of ingredients for every meal down to the last parsley leaf. Adjust the recipe ingredient amounts to your family's size and appetite for this two-meal program.

FRENCH LENTIL SOUP

Using the previous day's roast chicken and vegetables as the basis for your lentil soup means that most of your prep work is already done. To make soup, sort and rinse lentils and add to the soup pot. Add liquid and simmer. *C'est tout!* Paired meals work well when you prepare the more laborious meal on a non-work day when you have more time. The second meal requiring less preparation is prepared the following work day. If your left-over vegetables seem scant, add 2-4 stalks celery, chopped, and another 1-2 onions cut in eights to the soup pot.

Note: Never soak lentils before cooking, it can make them hard to digest. Lentils are high in protein. You can make a vegan meal version of this soup using only roasted vegetables and vegetable broth.

INGREDIENTS:

Chicken, vegetables, and cooking juices from previous night's meal

1/2 pound (1 cup) lentils, sorted and rinsed

1 quart water (or 2 cups water plus 2 cups chicken broth) heated

1/2 tsp. marjoram   1/2 tsp. oregano

1 Tbs. balsamic vinegar

METHOD:

Put the left-overs from your *Poulet en Cocotte* into a soup pot or large saucepan. Sort the lentils and rinse well. Add the lentils to the pot. Pour in hot liquid. Bring to a boil. Lower heat. Cook until lentils are tender. (About 1 hr.) Add more liquid if needed. Remove chicken bones from soup. Reheat. Just before serving, stir in the balsamic vinegar.

The French have many cooking *trucs*, tricks that save money (or effort) without sacrificing taste. One *truc* is to stir a little wine vinegar or balsamic vinegar into a stew or soup immediately before serving to give a "cooked in wine" taste. And it must be added at the last minute to have best results. When you calculate the difference in the cost of even a cup of *vin ordinaire* vs. that of a tablespoon of vinegar and multiply by even one recipe per week, you can see some real yearly savings.

VIANDE ROUGE JACQUES

French women are expert at taking a less-expensive cut of meat and —with clever seasonings and the proper cooking method—make it taste as flavorful and succulent as if prepared from the most expensive cut in the butcher shop. This recipe is the best thing I know to do with a not-very-tender cut of red meat. The recipe was given to my son by some West Virginia friends for roasting venison. A couple of years ago I discovered an almost identical recipe for lamb in a French cookbook. This recipe also works well for a less-expensive cut of beef.

INGREDIENTS:

Chuck roast (beef), lamb shoulder (bone removed), or venison roast

(about 2 1/2 to 3 1/2 lbs.)

20 cloves of garlic, peeled

1/4 cup extra virgin olive oil

2 tsp. curry powder

salt to taste

METHOD: Preheat oven to 350 degrees. Rinse and pat meat dry with a paper towel. Place in a 2-quart oven safe casserole with cover. With a sharp knife, cut 20 slits in the top of the meat. Tuck a clove of garlic into each slit. Pour the olive oil over the meat. Sprinkle on the curry powder and salt. Cover and bake for about 1 1/2 hours. Remove from the oven. Slice in 3/4 inch slices. Place broad side of meat slices in meat juices. Return to oven uncovered and continue to bake (checking every 10 minutes and toward the end, every 5 minutes) until the juices are absorbed into the meat and the meat has tenderized and browned. This additional baking usually takes about 30 to 45 minutes. Serve meat with brown rice and steamed spinach. Any left-over meat makes a wonderful sandwich with a whole grain bread and a good mustard. Shredded cabbage salad is good with the sandwiches.

BROWN RICE

Brown rice's taste and nutrition are so superior to those of white rice that I have almost given up eating white rice. Brown rice does require longer cooking time than white rice, however. I have been cooking brown rice (both long grain and short grain) for more than 45 years by this method; I always have wonderful rice. Allow at least an hour and fifteen minutes preparation time. I give you both a stove top and a microwave method. Cooked brown rice freezes well. I keep a container in the freezer to pair with stir fry or curry for a quick meal. Brown rice tastes wonderful with almost any meat and sauce dish. When you are trying to lose weight, brown rice is a wise substitute for wheat pastas.

INGREDIENTS:

   1 cup brown rice, well rinsed

   2 and 1/2 cups water

   1 tsp. salt

METHOD *for Stove Top*:

In a 2-quart pan with tight lid, put the 1 cup rinsed brown rice and 2 1/2 cups water at room temperature. Put the pan uncovered on the burner of the stove. Bring to boiling. Boil 5 minutes. Lower heat, cover pan, and simmer 45 minutes. If rice begins to scorch on bottom, add water. Never stir rice while cooking. At the end of 45 minutes, do not remove the lid. Turn off heat. Let rice stand covered 15 minutes. Fluff with a fork and serve.

METHOD *for Microwave*:

In a 2-quart microwavable casserole with tight-fitting lid, put salt, 1 cup rinsed brown rice and 2 and 1/2 cups water at room temperature. Cover. Microwave on HIGH power for 5 minutes. Then, microwave on 50% power for 45 minutes. Allow rice to stand covered for 15 minutes. Fluff with a fork and serve. Remember microwaves vary. You may need to adjust cooking time for your particular microwave.

PAN BAGNAT

Pan Bagnat (Provençal for bathed bread) is the ultimate chic French Riviera sandwich. The sandwich's taste secret is that the bread is bathed in rich olive oil and refrigerated under a weight that blends the flavors of the fish and vegetables. Oily and messy—but oh-so-delicious.!

INGREDIENTS:

1 baguette

2 - 4 Tbs. olive oil   5 garlic cloves, minced

4 medium tomatoes, peeled, seeded, sliced thinly

1 5-oz. can albacore tuna, drained

1 yellow or green sweet pepper, cut in thin circles

1 small mild, red onion, thinly sliced

1/4 cup black olives, thinly sliced   1 Tbs. capers

1 2-oz. can flat anchovy fillets

METHOD: Slice the baguette or loaf in half lengthwise. Spread the cut sides with olive oil. Mince the garlic and spread, pressing into the bread. On the bottom half of the sandwich, layer ingredients in the following order: tomatoes, tuna, sweet pepper, onion, black olives, capers, anchovy filets. Place the top on sandwich, cut into two portions, and wrap each portion tightly in plastic wrap. Place two portions side by side on a flat pan. Place a small cutting board on top of the sandwich portions. Put a weight on top of the cutting board.(A brick sealed in a Ziplock bag will do nicely.) Refrigerate 1 to 24 hours.

To serve, remove the plastic and cut in serving-sized portions. This is an oily sandwich to eat by hand. At the beach, you can wash off the oil in the sea. Eating *pan bagnat* in other locales, you may prefer to eat the sandwich open-faced with a knife and fork.

MARIA'S MIGAS

For a quick, light supper, the French might whip up an *omelette au fines herbes*. But in South Texas, a quick supper would more likely be *migas*. This recipe calls for *nopalitos*, pads of prickly pear cactus from which spines have been removed. Fresh is too much work, use prepared sold in glass jars. *Nopalitos* have a taste somewhere between a green bean and a green pepper. They are wonderfully low-calorie, low-fat, low sodium and exceptionally nutritious. If you can't find *nopalitos* in your market, substitute 1/2 cup cooked French-cut green beans or chopped Roma tomatoes. This recipe was shared with me by my friend Maria who makes delicious *migas*.

INGREDIENTS: (for one serving)

1 Tbs. olive oil   2 corn tortillas, torn into bite-size pieces

1/4 cup yellow onion, chopped

2 cloves garlic, peeled and minced

1/8 tsp. dried ground red pepper, NOT cayenne

1 cup canned *nopalitos*, drained and rinsed

2 eggs (*or* 1 egg plus 1 egg white), beaten

1 - 2 Tbs. grated cheese: *queso blanco*, mozzarella, or feta

salt to taste   salsa   chopped fresh cilantro leaves (optional)

METHOD: Put the *nopalito* pieces in a colander, rinse and let drain a few minutes. Heat a non-stick skillet. Add oil. When oil is hot, add the torn pieces of corn tortilla and cook until crispy. Lower heat and stir in onion, garlic, and pepper. Cook for several minutes to soften, stirring to prevent scorching. Add drained *nopalitos* to the tortilla pieces and onions. Stir into the mixture and cook several minutes Mixture should be hot all through when you add the eggs. Pour the beaten eggs evenly over the tortillas and vegetables. Add cheese and salt. Lower heat. Do not stir unless scorching. When almost set, fold the cooked mixture omelette style. Transfer to a plate. Top with salsa and cilantro.

COUSCOUS

This North African dish is as popular in Paris as Chinese cuisine in San Francisco. I learned this version of *couscous* from my Tunisian maid. Fatma would have been fired many times had I not realized that, if I sent her packing, I would never learn her secrets for making what I considered the best *couscous* in Tunisia. A robust olive oil is essential. Do not use cayenne. I use a mild "ground red pepper" from my natural foods store. This recipe uses chicken. *Couscous* is wonderful made with lamb. Beef is not bad. I never cared for the fish version. Pork? Don't even think about it.

INGREDIENTS:

2 lbs. chicken breasts and leg quarters

  (*or* 1 whole chicken, cut into serving pieces)

1/3 cup good grade olive oil

5 cloves garlic, peeled   1 yellow onion, cut in fourths

2 medium zucchini, cut in 2 in. pieces

4 carrots, scraped and cut into 3 in. pieces

4 stalks of celery, cut into 3 in. pieces

1 medium turnip, peeled and quartered

1 large potato, peeled and quartered

8 oz. winter squash or fresh pumpkin, cut in 2 in. cubes

1/4 cup cilantro leaves   1 Tbs. tomato puree or paste

1 cup cooked chickpeas

1/4 to 1/2 tsp. ground red pepper   1/4 tsp. black pepper

3/4 tsp. salt   1/2 tsp. dried thyme

1 cup water

10 or 12 green olives (be sure pits are removed)

1 cup *couscous*   1 cup chilled water

METHOD: Heat the olive oil in the bottom of a *couscousière* or a cooking pot large enough to hold the chicken and vegetables with several inches of space between top of ingredients and the top of pot. Brown the chicken pieces on all sides, several pieces at a time, until all are browned.

Return the chicken to the cooking pot. Add vegetables (except celery and zucchini), spices and water. Bring to a boil, and then lower temperature. Simmer for 20 minutes.

While stew simmers, put the *couscous* grains in a bowl and slowly add the cold water, a little at a time, tossing the grains lightly with a fork to help them absorb the liquid. Set the top section of the *couscousiére* onto the steaming pot. Carefully transfer moistened *couscous* grains into the top (steamer) section. Cover. (No *couscousiére*? See alternate instructions.) Several times during the steaming, skim oily broth from top of stew and sprinkle over the steaming grains. (This is tricky. Be careful not to burn yourself as you lift up the top of the *couscous* cooker to ladle the broth. Also, take care you do not cause too much of the *couscous* to fall through the steamer holes into the broth.) Add celery, zucchini, and chickpeas and green olives. Simmer an additional 20 minutes. Sprinkle broth over the *couscous* grains at least once during this last 20 minutes cooking time.

Alternate instructions for couscous: Follow instructions on the package of *couscous*. If no instructions are available, try this: Bring one cup water to a boil. Skim about 1/4 cup of the broth from the top of the cooking chicken and vegetable stew and add to the water. Stir in 1 cup of *couscous* grains. Cover and remove from the heat. Allow to stand 5 to 10 minutes. Toss lightly with a fork and follow serving instructions below.

To serve: Put the steamed *couscous* grains in a bowl and ladle an additional 1/3 to 1/2 cup of hot broth over the grains. Arrange the chicken and vegetables on top of the *couscous*. Serve the broth and chickpeas in a separate bowl.

CERTAIN AGE CHEESECAKE

Today, women of a "certain age" are encouraged to include soy in their diet to increase their intake of isoflavones. This dessert includes both tofu (soy curd) and soy milk. Be sure to use the soft-style tofu.

INGREDIENTS:

1 16-oz. pkg. soft-style tofu

3/4 cup soy milk (vanilla or plain)   1 egg

1 tsp. vanilla or almond extract (if using plain soy milk)

1 9-inch prepared crumb crust

METHOD:

Preheat oven to 375 degrees F. Drain the tofu and cut into 2-inch cubes. In a food processor or blender combine the tofu, milk, and egg. Process until smooth. (You can omit the egg; if so, decrease milk by 2 Tablespoons.) Pour the filling into the crumb crust. (Make sure your crumb crust is in an oven-safe pan.) Place the pie into the preheated oven and bake 40 to 50 minutes or until a knife tip inserted into the center of the pie comes out clean.   When done, remove the cheesecake from the oven and cool on a wire rack. To serve, cut a wedge and top with fresh or frozen fruit. For a sweeter dessert, sweeten fruit with sugar or stevia. Or you can sprinkle sugar, stevia, or your powdered sweetener of choice directly on the baked cheesecake.

Almost any fresh fruit or all-fruit jam makes a good topping for this cheesecake. Try fresh or frozen blueberries, raspberries, blackberries, cherries, kiwis or sliced mangoes. Fresh pineapple—or drained, canned pineapple— is delicious. A tablespoon of your favorite all-fruit jam is super easy. You can drizzle warm chocolate or caramel sauce over the cheesecake and top with chopped nuts or a teaspoon of warmed peanut butter. A lemon or orange custard sauce is elegant. You can sprinkle a teaspoon of Cointreau or other fruit liqueur over the top and garnish with whipped cream or whipped topping. Yogurt and fruit is good too.

SABLÉS

Many butter-heavy recipes originating in the north of France, become healthier (and more economical for us to prepare) when prepared as in other French regions where the cuisine uses little animal fat. Unless you make these cookies using imported French butter, you likely will not notice much difference in oil and butter versions. (I didn't—even using organic sweet cream butter in the test version.) These low-sugar, sandy-textured French *Sablés* (Sandies) can be varied with an assortment of flavorings. You can also make them with margarine—or with butter as they are traditionally made in Normandy.

INGREDIENTS:

7 fluid ounces (7/8 cup)extra light olive oil or canola oil

1/3 (or 1/2) cup sugar   1/4 tsp. salt

2 egg yolks

2 tsp. vanilla extract (strong extract use 1 tsp. + 1 tsp water)

2 cups unbleached flour

METHOD:

In a mixing bowl put all the ingredients except the flour. Mix well. Add flour. Stir until well blended. Divide the dough into 2 portions. Put each portion on a sheet of waxed paper about 12 inches long and form into a log about 8 inches long. Roll the paper around the dough logs and twist the ends. Refrigerate at least 1 hour before baking. To bake, while preheating the oven to 350 degrees F., slice the dough into coins 1/3 inch thick. Arrange on an oiled baking sheet 1 inch apart. Bake 18 - 20 minutes, until bottoms are nicely browned and edges are golden. Remove from oven and place baking sheet on wire rack. Allow *Sablés* to cool on the baking sheet.

Variations: For lemon *Sablés*, add the zest of one large lemon when mixing the sugar and oil. You can make a delicately-flavored tea biscuit substituting peach, strawberry, or raspberry flavoring oil in place of the vanilla. See flavoring oil's instructions for exact amount. Potency varies.

CHIC&SLIM JAM (CONFITURE)

You will usually find jars of homemade preserves (*confiture*) in a French kitchen. Surprising to many Americans, the French often prefer to make their homemade jams and preserves from dried rather than fresh fruits. Taste the more intensely-flavored jams made from dried fruit, and you will understand why. The French also prefer to use fruit juices instead of refined sugar for all or most of the sweetening in these jams. I love figs, apricots, and prunes. I make an easy microwave version of an all-fruit jam from each of them. Figs pair with white grape juice, apricots with apple juice, and prunes with red grape juice to make a very berry flavored jam. You would never believe this jam was made with prunes. The method for all these jams is the same. If you are not an experienced jam maker, see the instructions for testing jams in the jelly and jam section of any standard cookbook. You can also make these jams using traditional stovetop methods.

INGREDIENTS:

12 oz. (2 cups) dried fruit (figs, pitted prunes, *or* apricots)

1 cup water

1 12 oz. can of frozen juice concentrate (apple *or* grape)

1 lemon, thinly sliced (*or* juice of 1 lemon)

METHOD: Put dried fruit and water in a 2-quart microwave safe cooking dish. (A 2-quart Pyrex measuring container with handle works well.) Microwave on high for 10 minutes. Let stand 1 hour until fruit softens. Put the softened fruit and liquid into a blender or food processor and puree. Return the fruit puree to the microwave safe cooking container, add the juice concentrate. Cover and microwave on high, stirring at 5 minute intervals until the jam has thickened. Be sure to cover the pan. This jam bubbles and splatters as it cooks. Cooked uncovered, the jam will likely splatter and make a BIG mess in your microwave. When jam is sufficiently thickened, put the jam into sterilized jars and cover tightly. Refrigerate jam. Any jam that will not be used in a week should be frozen until time for use.

RESOURCES

BOOKS

French Chic: How To Dress Like A Frenchwoman (Villard Books 1988) Susan Sommers. An excellent book on how French women achieve their fantastic chic. A classic. Photos look dated, but the principles apply. *Note:* The author Susan Sommers is a fashion journalist and consultant. Do not confuse with Suzanne Somers, the actress and author of the weight loss books.

Audrey Style (HarperCollins 1999) Pamela Clarke Keogh. Like *French Chic*, this style biography of beloved actress Audrey Hepburn is an excellent resource for studying French chic. Audrey Hepburn's style was her own marvelous invention. But the principles behind that style were very French and much influenced by her favorite French designer Hubert de Givenchy.

Women&Beauty (William Morrow and Company 1984) Sophia Loren. The Italian-born actress wrote this book on mature beauty around age 50. Now, a quarter-century later, Sophia Loren's still-radiant beauty is excellent proof of the value of the techniques and philosophy in this book. Wonderful photos and much how-to advice.

Taking The Waters: Spirit, Art, Sensuality (Abbeville Press 1992) Alev Lytle Croutier. French women have long used various hydrotherapies to keep them chic and slim. This beautiful book is a wonderful source to learn about this delightful practice.

French Style (Clarkson N. Potter 1982) Susan Slesin, Stafford Cliff & Jacques Dirand. Many photos illustrate the book's excellent information on how the French decorate their homes.

French Tea: The Pleasures of the Table (Hearst Books 1993) Carole Manchester. The French enjoy afternoon tea, just as the English do. This book, illustrated with elegant photographs, shows teatime in a variety of French settings. Includes recipes for French pastries.

Le Divorce (Dutton 1997) Diane Johnson. Impossible to truly feel sympathy for any of the characters in this award-winning novel. But the book provides good insights into French life. Much information about French women.

And God Created The French (Robert Davies 1998) Louis-Bernard Robitaille. An entertaining look at the French, particularly Parisians. The author's profiles of Catherine Deneuve, Isabelle Adjani, and Françoise Giroud give good insights into French women.

French Toast: An American in Paris Celebrates the Maddening Mysteries of the French (St. Martin's Press 1999) Harriet Welty Rochefort. Another good profile of life in Paris. Wonderful portrait of French women in late 1990s.

Anne Barone's other Chic & Slim Books:

Chic & Slim: how those chic French women eat all that rich food and still stay slim

Chic & Slim Techniques: 10 techniques to make you chic & slim à la française

Chic & Slim Toujours: aging beautifully like those chic French women

Purchase information for these and other books by Anne Barone on *annebarone.com*.

AUDIOTAPES VIDEOTAPES DVDS

Weight Loss (Time Warner AudioBooks 1997) Belleruth Naparstek. The best audio tape I have found to help you lose weight. Particularly good for those who have a problem with body image and who need motivation for regular exercise.

French Kiss (1995) Meg Ryan and Kevin Kline. This comedy presents a wonderful comparison of French and American women, as well as lessons in how French women handle men. You also see a good demonstration of the art of the French pout.

Denise Austin Mat Workout Based on the Work of J.H. Pilates (Artisan) Good explanation of the Pilates method precedes the first 20-minute mat workout's excellent stretching and toning exercises. Second workout is her *Yoga Essentials* on speed. Not recommended. If you are familiar with Denise Austin's early videos, you can see how Pilates and Yoga have slimmed her bulky muscles. Less annoying chatter than usual for Denise.

The Method Pilates: Precision Toning and Sculpting (PPI Entertainment) Jennifer Kries brings the dignity of the classically trained dancer to this excellent toning and sculpting tape. This program makes my body feel so good that I look forward to the sessions. Uses hand weights.

Buns of Steel Step 2000 (Maier Group) Workout lead by Tamilee Webb. I bought this exercise video used on eBay more than a decade ago. Still my favorite cold weather indoor exercise workout. Uses an exercise step. Aerobic as well as great toning for buns and legs.

CHIC & SLIM LE WEBSITE
annebarone.com

This companion website for Anne Barone's *Chic & Slim* books offers frequently updated articles, tips, links, recipes, and other resources to help you eat all that rich food and still stay slim the way chic French women do. On *annebarone.com* you will also find reader comments on how *Chic & Slim* has worked for others. You can send your own *Chic & Slim* success stories there too. I look forward to hearing from you.

NOTES ON SOURCES

Introduction: *Making the Case for Yourself: A Diet Book For Smart Women* by Susan Estrich, Putnam Publishing Group 1998—*Dr. Susan Love's Hormone Book* by Susan M. Love, Random House 1997.

Chapter 1: "Person with oldest verifiable age dies in France at 122" by Craig R. Whitney of *The New York Times News Service*. 1997—"On Wine, Women, and the Art of the Kiss"by Marianne Jacobbi. *European Travel & Life*, April 1992—"Parlez-vous Francais?" by Dave Barry Syndicated column read on *www.sacbee.com* (Sacramento Bee) 16 August 1998—Knight Ridder article by Brigid Schulte in October 1997—"Katell Le Bourhis" *Elle Decor* 1999.

Chapter 2: *The Second Sex* by Simone de Beauvoir, Bantam Books 1961— "Paris Fax: When It Comes to Love, 50 Million French Women Can't Be Wrong." by Carolyn White. *Elle*. February 1994—*Elegance* by Genevieve Antoine Dariaux, Doubleday 1964—*French Toast* by Harriet Welty Rochefort, St. Martin's Press 1999—*Superchic: Reporting on Fashion* by James Brady, Little, Brown & Company 1974—"Metropolitan Diary" by Enid Nemy, *The New York Times*, August 1999—"The Revolutionist's Handbook" Four Plays by Bernard Shaw, Washington Square Press.

Chapter 3: *Use The Right Word: A Modern Guide to Synonyms* edited by S. I. Hayakawa, Reader's Digest Association 1968—"French Polish: Small dogs, the shortest of skirts and steely discipline" by Alicia Drake *British Vogue* November 1998—"Japanese tourists at the Louvre" by Suzy Menkes *International Herald Tribune* 1998.

Chapter 4: *Low Fat Lies: High Fat Frauds and the healthiest diet in the world* by Dr. Mary Flynn and Dr. Kevin Vigilante (Lifeline Press) as reported in *The New York Times* article 25 May 1999—Laura Fraser article in a *Salon. com* article 2000 about Paul Rozin research—"The European Weight-Loss Syndrome" in *Allure* Brochure—William R. Clark in *A Means to An End: The Biological Basis of Aging and Death*, Oxford University Press 1999—*Encore Provence: New Adventures in the South of France* by Peter Mayle Alfred A. Knopf 1999—"Susan Powter" by Jan Jarboe, *Texas Monthly* November 1993—*The*

Physiology of Taste by Brillat-Savarin, Translated by M.F.K. Fisher, Knopf 1971—"Eternal Woman" By Anne-Marie O'Neill, Julie Jordon and Cathy Nolan People 31 May 1999—*The Art of Living Consciously* by Dr. Nathaniel Branden, Simon & Schuster 1997

Chapter 5: "Paris Kiosque: Paris Quick Takes" by Harriet Welty Rochefort The Paris Pages at *www.paris.org* March 1997—*Eagle's Nest* by John Ruskin 1872—*Not For Packrats Only: How to Clean Up, Clear Out, and Dejunk Your Life Forever!* by Don Aslett, Penguin 1991—"Postscript" by Grace Deer *Sedona* Magazine Spring 1997—"Wired At Heart" by Leslie Bennetts *Vanity Fair* November 1997—"No Satisfaction: The trials of the shopping nation" by John Cassidy *The New Yorker*—*Our Enemy, the Customer* by Simone Barbaras 1995—*French Style* By Suzanne Slesin, Stafford Cliff, and Jacques Dirand Clarkson N. Potter 1982—Gary Kamiya in "A Brief History of Salons" article on *Salon.com*—Thomas Friedman editorial on the real Y2K disease in *The New York Times* January 2000—*The Tea Lover's Treasury* by James Norwood Pratt 101 Productions 1982—Quote on Elizabeth Hurley from January *Elle* article, profile on EH—*And God Created The French* by Louis-Bernard Robitaille—Belleruth Naparstek's *Weight Loss* audiotape

Chapter 6: Ohio State University study reported in the *Corpus Christi Caller-Times* 31 August, 1998—"Your Attitudes" relating information about the marriage study by Dr. Sandra Murray—"Domestic Violence Viewpoint" by Nancy B. Mahon appeared in *Corpus Christi Caller-Times* 28 Ocober 1998—*The Argument Culture* by Deborah Tannen Random House 1998—*The New York Times Book Review*: The Argument Culture by Larissa MacFarquhar, quoted on the *Amazon.com* catalog page for *The Argument Culture*—*Thrones, Dominations* by Dorothy L. Sayers and Jill Paton Walsh, St. Martin's Press 1998—"Strangers In the Night" by Christine Schoeffer *Salon.com* 15 Feb. 2000—"Savoir Faire: Going Solo" by Kristin Hohenadel. *Paris Notes* June 1997—*Acquired Tastes* by Peter Mayle Bantam Books 1992—"After Five Decades, A Spy Tells Her Tale" by David Ignatius. *The Washington Post*, 28 December 1998 —"Durex Global Sex Survey" By Rose DeWolf reported in the Knight Ridder newspapers 25 September 1998.

MERCI BEAUCOUP

My commitment to share with you the *Chic&Slim* philosophy has never faltered. Still, there have been difficult moments as I persevered to create the books and to create and maintain the *Chic&Slim* website. These are fundamentally solo operations. Yet I could not have continued to devote my full time to them, nor would they have been as effective, without support and help from friends and family.

As always, I am most grateful to my son John. His efforts on behalf of Anne Barone's *Chic&Slim* are so extensive that I assure you that there would be neither book nor website without him. My Padre Island friends Sheryl & Bob White see that I remain alive and well. Bob's expertise in things automotive and computer are invaluable. I am also grateful to Betty Buchanan who has been such a supportive friend during my time on the Texas Riviera. Teresa & Ray Rabalais provided me with a wonderful place to live and work. My mother, Helen, made her guest room available for *Encore's* editing, typesetting, and cover design. Marsi Buckmelter's copyediting skills greatly improved the manuscript. Virginia Bandremer corrected my French. Marsi and Virginia, along with Marina Borough, Frances Ruiz, and others, read and provided comments and suggestions on improving *Chic&Slim Encore,* this second book in the *Chic & Slim* series.

To all those who shared recipes with me through the years, and especially to all of you *Chic&Slim Women* who have shared your knowledge and experiences, sent tips on articles and other resources, your contributions have been greatly appreciated. That is why I dedicated this book to you. *Merci Beaucoup.*

AU REVOIR

Good food is such joy! Dressing chic is such fun!

French women demonstrate that we can enjoy the good foods we love and still stay slim. They show us that we can easily maintain a chic, attractive personal style, even on the tightest budget. With *Chic&Slim ENCORE* you can dress as chic and stay as slim as French women—no matter where you live.

Success tip: Make changes in your eating, in your personal style, and in your lifestyle *gradually*.

If something does not seem right for you, or makes you uncomfortable, skip it. Try another technique. There are no "have-tos" in my French-inspired *Chic&Slim* system. Make your own choices about which of the available techniques for chic and slim are best for *you*.

Most important, make the process of losing weight, staying slim, and refining your own chic personal style a pleasure. Chic French women do. You can too! *Bonne chance.*

ANNE BARONE

CPSIA information can be obtained at www.ICGtesting.com
Printed in the USA
LVOW131009200612

286904LV00003B/95/P